CONTENTS

Introduction

Abortion is the seventy-first volume in the **Issues** series. The aim of this series is to offer up-to-date information about important issues in our world.

Abortion examines the arguments for and against abortion.

The information comes from a wide variety of sources and includes:
Government reports and statistics
Newspaper reports and features
Magazine articles and surveys
Web site material
Literature from lobby groups
and charitable organisations.

It is hoped that, as you read about the many aspects of the issues explored in this book, you will critically evaluate the information presented. It is important that you decide whether you are being presented with facts or opinions. Does the writer give a biased or an unbiased report? If an opinion is being expressed, do you agree with the writer?

Abortion offers a useful starting-point for those who need convenient access to information about the many issues involved. However, it is only a starting-point. At the back of the book is a list of organisations which you may want to contact for further information.

*****

Abortion

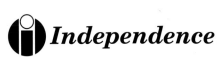

Independence

Educational Publishers
Cambridge

First published by Independence
PO Box 295
Cambridge CB1 3XP
England

© Craig Donnellan 2003

British Library Cataloguing in Publication Data
Abortion – (Issues Series)
I. Donnellan, Craig II. Series
363.4'6

ISBN 1 86168 253 0

Printed in Great Britain
MWL Print Group Ltd

Typeset by
Claire Boyd

Cover
The illustration on the front cover is by
Pumpkin House.

Abortion – the facts

Information from Brook Advisory Centres

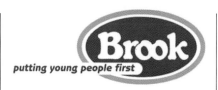

First things first

Abortion means ending a pregnancy so that it does not result in the birth of a child. If a woman thinks she is pregnant but hasn't had a pregnancy test done, she needs to do so as soon as possible.

What is a legal abortion?

In England, Wales and Scotland abortion is legal under 24 weeks of pregnancy if two doctors agree that it is necessary for one of the following reasons:

- having the baby would harm the woman's mental or physical health more than having the abortion. This involves the woman explaining how she feels about the pregnancy to a doctor.
- having the baby would harm the mental or physical health of any children she already has.

An abortion is also legal at any time in pregnancy if two doctors agree that:

- the abortion is necessary to save the woman's life or prevent serious permanent harm to her mental or physical health, or
- there is a high risk that the baby would be seriously handicapped.

Note that the stage of pregnancy is calculated from the first day of the woman's last period. Note also that different laws apply outside England, Wales and Scotland.

How can a woman get an abortion?

To get an abortion on the NHS, a woman needs to be referred by a doctor. This can be her own GP, or a doctor at a local family planning clinic or Brook Centre (for under-25s).

If a doctor has a moral objection to abortion, s/he does not have to be involved. However, s/he should explain this to their patient and make arrangements for her to see another doctor.

It is important to act quickly. The earlier a woman decides to have an abortion, the easier it is to get a free abortion on the NHS. Although the normal legal limit for abortion is 24 weeks, it is usually easiest to get an abortion on the NHS if a woman is under 12 weeks pregnant. There is an average of 2-4 weeks' waiting time on the NHS, so it is easier if a woman is under 8 weeks pregnant.

Women can refer themselves for a private abortion. Early abortions start from around £350 and go up to £750 or above in the later stages. For more information on private abortions, visit our useful organisations section.

Once referred for an NHS or private abortion, the woman will need to attend a consultation at the clinic. Her medical history will be taken and a nurse or doctor will discuss what will happen.

Under-16s

A young woman under 16 can have an abortion but special rules apply about consent. Brook Centres are used to seeing young people under 16 and can provide confidential help.

How are abortions carried out?

There are two main early abortion methods:

Medical abortion (known as 'the abortion pill')

Medical abortion can be performed in the first 9 weeks of pregnancy. It does not involve any surgery. The woman is given a pill (mifepristone) and 36 to 48 hours later, a tablet (prostaglandin) is placed in her vagina. These two drugs end most early pregnancies within the following four hours. It feels like having a heavy and rather painful period.

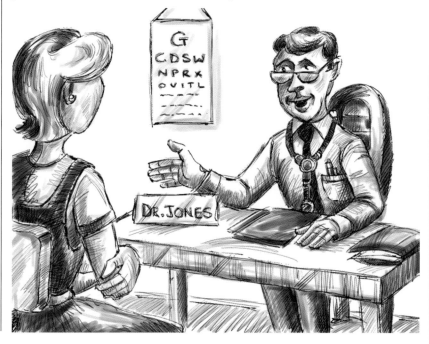

This method is not available everywhere. Women should check with the referring doctor whether this method is available on the NHS in their area.

Vacuum aspiration (known as 'the suction method')

This method is available up to 13 weeks of pregnancy. For this procedure the woman has either a general or local anaesthetic. The abortion is carried out through the vagina and there is no wound or stitches. The cervix (the entrance to the womb at the top of the vagina) is gently stretched to allow a tube to pass through it into the womb. Once the tube is inserted, it only takes a minute to remove the pregnancy by suction. Healthy women take only an hour or so to recover and most go home the same day.

Methods used for later abortions will depend on the stage of pregnancy. The exact procedure will be explained by a doctor or nurse before the abortion goes ahead.

Having an abortion should not affect a woman's ability to have a child in the future.

After an abortion

The woman will experience some bleeding for a few days after the abortion and may have pain like 'period pains'. Advice will be given on how to reduce the risk of infection.

If bleeding or pain is severe, or she has a raised temperature or unusual vaginal discharge, she should see a doctor as soon as possible as this could mean that she has an infection which needs treatment.

The woman will need to see a doctor about one to six weeks after the abortion to make sure all is well.

It is possible to become pregnant again as soon as 7 days after an abortion. So the woman needs to think about future contraception.

■ The above information is from Brook Advisory Centres' web site which can be found at www.brook.org.uk

© Brook Advisory Centres

Public opinions

Arguments for and against abortion

People often have strong views about abortion. These are some of the arguments used to justify legal abortion, or to oppose it.

The arguments against legal abortion

■ Human life begins at conception and abortion destroys respect for human life.
■ Abortion is a violent act that damages a mother and her baby. It is uncivilised and unjust.
■ There are alternatives to abortion, such as adoption.
■ Abortion damages women because they suffer post-abortion guilt and trauma.
■ Abortion is rarely necessary to save the life of the woman.
■ Abortion encourages brutality towards children and child abuse.
■ Abortion on grounds of fetal abnormality encourages discrimination against disabled people.

The arguments for legal abortion

■ The embryo or fetus should be respected as potential human life but does not have the same value as a born person.
■ Women are capable of making

British Pregnancy Advisory Service

the right moral choices and can follow their own consciences.

■ A pregnant woman understands her own personal circumstances better than anyone else and so is in the best position to know whether she should or should not have a child.
■ Legal abortion is relatively safe and is likely to cause a woman less harm than forcing her to continue her pregnancy and have an unwanted child.
■ It is better for children to be born to parents who want and love them.
■ It is not possible to prevent unwanted pregnancies by contraception alone.
■ Public opinion supports legal abortion.
■ When abortion is illegal women tend to travel elsewhere because they are so desperate to avoid having to continue an unwanted pregnancy.

What is the alternative?

There is no practical alternative to easily accessible legal abortion. If the law denied abortion to women with unplanned pregnancies then they would either travel to places where they could obtain legal abortions or they would seek illegal procedures in this country as they did before 1967.

Some women, possibly tens of thousands each year, would become mothers of unplanned, unwanted children. This would have major consequences for individual women, for public health and for society as a whole. Therefore it is not in the interests of individual women or society to turn the clock back.

Public opinion on abortion

Public opinion in Great Britain and Northern Ireland supports legal abortion.

A MORI poll commissioned in February 1997 by BPAS and Birth Control Trust showed that 64 per cent of those asked agreed with the statement 'Abortion should be made legally available for all who want it', while 25 per cent disagreed. The proportion of British adults who agreed with the statement had increased by 10 per cent since 1980, while the proportion that disagreed had fallen by 11 per cent.

Religious positions on abortion

Roman Catholic

The Roman Catholic Church holds the view that life begins at the moment of conception and should be protected from this time. In 1869 Pope Pius VI declared that ensoulment takes place at conception and since then this has been restated frequently in documents expressing the official church teaching.

Church of England

The Church of England holds the view that all human life is created by God and should be nurtured, supported and protected. This principle applies to both the mother and the fetus therefore the Church recognises the need for a balance between compassion for the mother and responsibility for the life of the fetus. In 1983 the General Synod passed a resolution that recognised that 'in situations where the continuance of the pregnancy threatens the life of the mother, a termination of pregnancy may be justified and that there must be adequate and safe provision in our society for such situations'.

Church of Scotland

In 1988 the Church of Scotland Board of Social Responsibility recommended that abortion be permitted 'on grounds that the continuance of the pregnancy would involve serious risk to the life or present great danger to the health, whether physical or mental, of the pregnant woman'.

Jewish

Judaism permits abortion if the mother's life is at risk through continuing the pregnancy, which includes the risk of suicide.

Muslim

Islam holds the view that abortion is permitted in extreme circumstances such as when the mother's life is endangered. Some Islamic scholars would also sanction abortion if the pregnancy was the result of rape. Abortion is seen as more acceptable if it takes place before 120 days when it is believed the soul enters the fetus.

Hindu

Hinduism traditionally forbids abortion except for serious medical reasons.

Buddhism

Buddhists are free to act according to their own insights and understanding, at the same time Buddhism teaches that people should act responsibly. They undertake to cultivate an attitude of loving kindness (metta) and compassion (karuna) to living things.

Humanism

Humanism is not a religion but a system of ethical beliefs based on the view that humans should take responsibility for their own lives and show concern for the quality of life of others. Tolerance and open-mindedness are valued. Humanists believe that human life should be valued but do not believe that there is a clear point at which a fetus becomes a person. Humanists believe that there are no moral grounds for refusing an abortion in early pregnancy and even in late pregnancy abortion may be 'the humane and moral choice'. Official church teaching on abortion does not necessarily influence the decisions women make. It is common for Catholics to disagree with church teaching on abortion and abortion is common in many Catholic countries.

What does BPAS believe about abortion?

BPAS believes that abortion should be legal and that women should be free to decide if, and when, they have children. Those who oppose abortion are a minority. They are entitled to their views and values but they should respect the views and values of others.

Better sex education and improved contraceptive services would help women avoid unwanted pregnancy but would not eliminate the need for abortion entirely. Contraception is not 100 per cent effective and a planned pregnancy may become a problem.

Abortion is an essential part of health care and should be freely available to all women through a publicly funded NHS.

Abortion can be a responsible choice. It has no fewer morals than the decision to have a child.

■ The above information is from British Pregnancy Advisory Service's web site which can be found at www.bpas.org Alternatively, see page 41 for their address details.

© British Pregnancy Advisory Service (BPAS)

Opinions on abortion

Abortion should be made legally available for all that want it

Agree very strongly	15%
Agree strongly	15%
Agree	34%
Neither agree nor disagree	9%
Disagree	13%
Disagree strongly	5%
Disagree very strongly	7%
Don't know	2%

Circumstances when people approve or disapprove of abortion

	Approve	Disapprove	Don't know
When the woman's life is in danger	93%	3%	4%
When the woman's health is at risk	88%	6%	6%
In a case of rape	88%	6%	6%
When the child would have a mental disability	67%	20%	13%
When the child would have a physical disability	66%	21%	13%
When the woman was under 16	58%	29%	13%

Source: British Pregnancy Advisory Service

Abortion statistics

Information from the British Pregnancy Advisory Service (BPAS)

In 2000 there were 175,542 abortions performed on women resident in England and Wales.

How the number and rate of abortions has changed

From 1968 to 1973, the annual numbers of legal abortions for women living in England and Wales increased rapidly and then levelled off at about 100,000 a year. Abortion numbers then rose each year until 1991, mainly because the numbers of women in the population aged 15 to 44 (the fertile ages) grew due to a large increase in the birth rate in Britain between 1956 and 1963. There were more abortions between 1975 and 1990 because there were more women to become pregnant. A further factor in the rise in the number of abortions was the fall in the popularity of marriage among young women. Unmarried women are more likely to have an abortion if they have an unplanned pregnancy. The number of abortions has remained stable between 1998 and 2000. Reasons for this new stability could be due to abortion becoming a more acceptable solution than ever before when contraception fails or women fail to use it properly.

The number of abortions in England and Wales declined between 1990 and 1995, and better use of contraception is likely to have been an important factor in this. There was a 7 per cent increase in the number of abortions in 1996, largely due to the effects of a Pill scare in 1995 about the safety of certain brands of oral contraceptives. This undermined the confidence of many women in hormonal methods of contraception and decreased their use. The abortion rate has continued to rise, possibly because of continued concern about the safety of contraceptive hormones, especially among young women, and possibly because abortion is seen by more women as an acceptable way to manage an unwanted pregnancy. The increased

British Pregnancy Advisory Service

Numbers and rates of abortions carried out on residents of England and Wales for the last 5 years

Year	Number	Rate
1996:	167,916	or 16.00
1997:	170,145	or 16.30
1998:	177,871	or 17.13
1999:	173,701	or 16.79
2000:	175,542	or 16.94

per 1000 women aged 15-44

abortion rate in 1996 was widely publicised and may have educated women that abortion is a legal and safe choice.

Who pays for abortions?

Unlike maternity services when a woman wants to continue a pregnancy, abortions are not automatically available through the NHS. On average, throughout England and Wales the NHS pays for approximately three-quarters (74.9 per cent) of abortions. There are significant differences between

regions. In some areas the NHS pays for more than 90 per cent of abortions, in other regions it pays for less than 50 per cent. Statistics are published annually by the Office of National Statistics showing the contribution of each health authority to the funding of abortions in their area.

At what gestation do most abortions occur?

Almost 90 per cent of abortions are in the first 12 weeks of pregnancy. Just 1.5 per cent are after 20 weeks.

Abortions in England and Wales 2000 by gestation (total 175,542)

Under 9 weeks:	75,908	43.2%
9-12 weeks:	79,000	45.0%
13-19 weeks:	18,079	10.3%
20 weeks and over:	2,555	1.5%

Later abortions are often for the following reasons:

- The woman may not have been able to get a hospital appointment earlier in the pregnancy;
- she may not have realised she was pregnant (this is more common with young women and women approaching the meno-

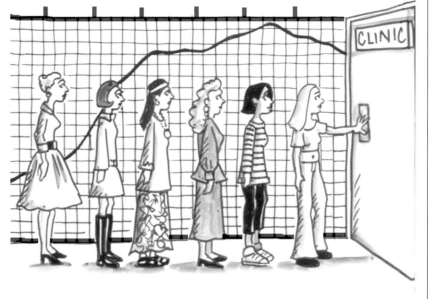

1950 1960 1970 1980 1990 2000

pause both of whom may have infrequent periods);

- very young women may feel unable to cope and so hide the pregnancy;
- sometimes the pregnancy was originally wanted but the woman's circumstances change (perhaps because she is abandoned by her partner or finds that her parents are not willing to provide her with a home or any other support);
- fetal abnormality is an important reason for late abortion, as many cannot be diagnosed early in pregnancy.

At what age do women have abortions?

Abortions in England and Wales 2000 by age (total 175,542)

Under 16	3,748	2.1%
16-19	33,218	18.9%
20-24	47,099	26.8%
25-29:	37,852	21.6%
30-34:	28,735	16.4%
35-44:	24,383	13.9%
45 and over:	459	–
Not stated:	48	–

The highest number of abortions is among women aged 20-24. However, a great deal of attention has been focused on teenagers because England and Wales has one of the highest teenage pregnancy rates for 15- 19-year-olds in Western Europe.

One woman in five who has an abortion is married; many others are in stable relationships. Abortion is not only an issue for single women. 47 per cent of women who have abortions have at least one child already.

Why do women from abroad travel to Britain for abortion?

In 2000 almost 10,000 women who lived abroad travelled to England to have an abortion.

Most of these women came from other parts of the British Isles, mainly from Northern Ireland (1,528) and the Irish Republic (6,391). Those from elsewhere in the world came because abortion is available in their countries only up to 12 weeks (France and Italy) or not available at all (the Arab states), or to ensure complete confidentiality.

The numbers have fallen from their peak of 57,000 in 1973 because most other European countries now have abortion laws that are less restrictive than those in Britain.

The reality of Irish abortion:
Facts and stats
BPAS has provided the ifpa with access to data detailing age, gestation and area of residence for the 8,214 Irish clients to whom it has provided abortion services since January 1997.

In 2000 almost 10,000 women who lived abroad travelled to England to have an abortion. Most of these women came from other parts of the British Isles, mainly from Northern Ireland

---

BPAS statistics analysed by the ifpa reveal the following key headline facts:

39.5% of all Irish clients, since January 1997, have self-referred, indicating that they have not availed of counselling in Ireland before travelling. While this figure is still high it does show that 60% have accessed some form of counselling.

79.5% of all Irish clients, since January 1997, have had their abortion at 12 weeks' gestation or less. UK Office for National Statistics (ONS) figures for 1996 indicate that this figure was 73% that year.

3.5% of all Irish clients, since January 1997, have had their abortion at 20 weeks' gestation or more.

- The above information is from British Pregnancy Advisory Service's (BPAS) web site which can be found at www.bpas.org Alternatively, see page 41 for their address details.

© *British Pregnancy Advisory Service (BPAS)*

Facts and statistics

Age at time of abortion, BPAS clients January 1997 to June 2000

Age Group	1997	1998	1999	Jan to June 2000	Total
<16	21	19	12	1	53 (0.64%)
16-19	379	422	386	172	1359 (16.41%)
20-24	854	925	933	379	3091 (37.32%)
25-34	768	868	883	354	2873 (34.69%)
35-44	273	261	236	102	872 (10.53%)
45+	10	9	10	4	33 (0.39%)
Total	2305	2504	2460	1012	8281

Gestation at time of abortion, BPAS clients January 1997 to June 2000

Weeks of gestation	1997	1998	1999	Jan to June 2000	Total
Nfs	1	3	4	1	9
<9	785	697	731	301	2514 (30.36%)
9-12	1086	1257	1187	493	4023 (48.58%)
13-14	171	217	190	81	659 (7.95%)
15-16	99	115	134	42	390 (4.7%)
17-19	99	128	119	45	391 (4.72%)
20+	64	87	95	49	295 (3.56%)
Total	2305	2504	2460	1012	8281

Source: British Pregnancy Advisory Service (BPAS)

All about abortions

Or everything you want to know about abortions but were afraid to ask

Most important fact: nobody, absolutely nobody likes having an abortion, and many abortions are avoidable by using the 'emergency contraceptive pill' within 72 hours of having unprotected sexual intercourse. Not using emergency contraception if you are worried that you could be pregnant, is 'burying your head in the sand' and hoping for the best. Get down to your family doctor, or any other family doctor, or your local family planning clinic or your local 'emergency room' NOW and get yourself the 'emergency contraceptive pill'.

Facts about abortions

There are few subjects which raise more emotion in people than that of abortion. The arguments rage backwards and forwards from 'it is murder' to 'it is the right of every woman to have an abortion if she wants one'.

These arguments all have some truth in them, but dealing with the facts:

- Abortion of foetuses up to the 24th week of pregnancy is legal in England, Scotland and Wales (in Northern Ireland it is only legal in exceptional circumstances)
- Abortion is available in these countries subject to the approval of two doctors
- 180,000 legal abortions are carried out in Britain every year
- The majority of abortions are carried out before 12 weeks

Further facts are:

- Legal abortion is very safe for the pregnant woman, and there is very little risk, particularly during early pregnancy
- Legal abortion does not normally interfere with you having a baby later on in life
- Legal abortion is free on the National Health Service in England, Scotland and Wales

If you're thinking about having an abortion

You'll need to think carefully about:

- Your moral stance on abortion
- Your religious stance (if any)
- How far pregnant you are (if you choose an abortion, the earlier you have one the better – before 12 weeks if possible)
- Where you are with your education at the present time
- The nature of the relationship that you have with your sexual partner
- Your age
- What your financial situation is – are you still living with your parents etc.
- The attitude of your parents and how supportive they will be whatever you decide (though you may choose not to tell them)

Whatever you decide there'll be ups and downs

You may, if you decide to have an abortion, have your baby adopted, or keep your baby, feel sad afterwards. This doesn't mean that you made the wrong decision – it is just that there are no absolute rights or wrongs in all this and whichever you decide there are upsides and downsides. You may:

- think that it is all right to have an abortion, but when it comes to it, find it hard to go through with
- think that abortion is all wrong, but when it comes to it, having an abortion is the better option

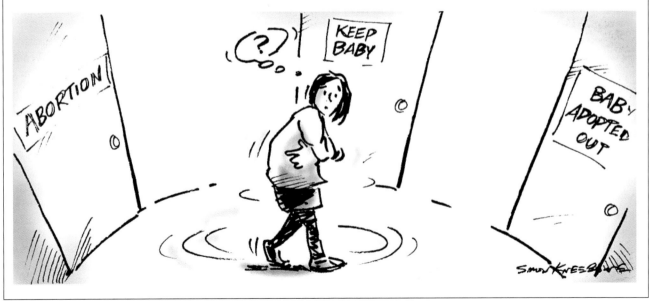

Grounds on which abortion is permitted in some countries

Country	To save the woman's life	To preserve physical health	To preserve mental health	Rape or incest reasons	Foetal impairment	Economic or social reasons	On request[1]
Austria	✓	✓	✓	✓	✓	✓	✓
Belgium[2]	✓	✓	✓	✓	✓	✓	✓
Denmark	✓	✓	✓	✓	✓	✓	✓
France[2]	✓	✓	✓	✓	✓	✓	✓
Germany[2]	✓	✓	✓	✓	✓	✓	✓
Ireland	✓	✗	✗	✗	✗	✗	✗
Italy[2]	✓	✓	✓	✓	✓	✓	✓
Netherlands	✓	✓	✓	✓	✓	✓	✓
Norway	✓	✓	✓	✓	✓	✓	✓
Spain	✓	✓	✓	✓	✓	✗	✗
Sweden	✓	✓	✓	✓	✓	✓	✓
United Kingdom	✓	✓	✓	✗	✓	✓	✗

1 For the purpose of this table, an abortion authorised on request is an abortion that is authorised in each of the other grounds within the same gestational limits, even if the law does not specifically mention such a ground.

2 The abortion laws in these countries require a woman seeking an abortion to state that she is in a condition of distress or a similar situation, depending on the country. The decision to have an abortion, however, is entirely the woman's.

Source: International Planned Parenthood Federation (IPPF)

Who to talk to

If you want to find out about getting an abortion (even if you don't really think that you want to go through it):

- You need to see a doctor, a general practitioner or someone from a charitable abortion clinic like the 'Pregnancy Advisory Service' or the 'Family Planning' service
- If the first doctor you see is not sympathetic about you having an abortion, don't be put off, but arrange to see another doctor without delay. You have the right to consult another family doctor under these circumstances
- The first doctor will then refer you on to a second doctor, either at a local hospital or someone who is part of the abortion clinic set-up

The laws about having an abortion

- Abortions must be carried out in a hospital or a clinic approved by the Department of Health such as those run by Marie Stopes International or the British Pregnancy Advisory Service
- Up to 24 weeks of pregnancy a woman who wants a safe abortion can have one legally with the agreement of two doctors
- These two doctors need to agree that your abortion is necessary for your mental and/or physical health
- It is not legal to have an abortion in Northern Ireland other than in the most exceptional of circumstances
- A legal abortion after 24 weeks of pregnancy is extremely rare and can only take place if the mother's life is in serious danger from the pregnancy or if there is something seriously wrong with the baby

The methods of 'abortion' that are used:

The abortion pill:

- This works for up to 9 weeks after the date that you had your last period
- It involves two or three visits to the clinic or hospital
- You take tablets given to you by the clinic or hospital at the first visit
- Two days later you visit again and have prostaglandin pessary (tablet) inserted into your vagina. You stay in hospital for a few hours after this until you have aborted, which sometimes involves having strong pains like period pains
- For a small number of people (less than one in twenty) this method does not work and you have to have the suction method described below

The suction, or vacuum aspiration, method:

- This can be used up to 12 weeks after you have had your last period
- You normally will be 'put out' by having a general anaesthetic, which may, when you come round from it, make you feel tired for a bit
- You don't normally have to stay in the clinic or hospital overnight

Both these methods are very safe and are unlikely to lead to any complications like not being able to have a baby later on.

For late abortions after 12 weeks:

- after 13 to 14 weeks different methods of abortion are used
- over 13 weeks there is a similar method as the abortion pill method but with some variation, and there may be more pain and bleeding
- another method is dilating your cervix under anaesthetic and sucking out the foetal remains

Remember

If you think that might be pregnant, and think that you want to have an abortion – act straight away – don't wait – because the earlier that you have an abortion, the safer and easier it is.

You can get pregnant again two weeks after you have had an abortion, so that even if sex is the last thing you are thinking of, make sure you get some decent advice about contraception

- The above information is from www.teenagehealthfreak.org

Common questions on abortion answered

If you are pregnant and do not want the baby then there is a lot to consider, a doctor and counsellors will do their best to advise you. However, here are a few of the common questions about abortion answered.

How late in a pregnancy can an abortion be done?
An abortion should be done as early as possible. Most abortions are done during the first 12 weeks of pregnancy because they are safest then. Sometimes abortions are done as late as 20 weeks, but this is very rare.

How safe is an abortion?
According to the experts 'Abortions are very safe. They are now one of the safest operations of all. And, the earlier the abortion, the lower the chance of any complications.'

If I have an abortion can I still have children later on?
Yes. Women who have an early abortion are just as likely as women in general to have a healthy baby in the future.

Is an abortion painful?
Local or general anaesthetic are used before an abortion to control pain. Most women feel cramps (like strong period cramps) for a short time. If a woman needs it, the doctor will give her extra medication for any pain.

How do you feel after an abortion?
In general, women consider abortion because being pregnant at that time is in some way wrong for them. Most women feel relief after their abortion and feel that they have made the right decision for themselves.

According to the experts 'Abortions are very safe. They are now one of the safest operations of all. And, the earlier the abortion, the lower the chance of any complications.'

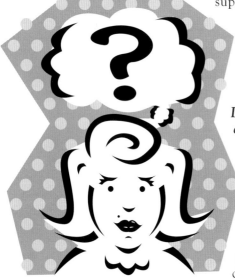

Some women feel sad or emotional afterwards due to the whole experience. You may need a supportive friend, relative or counsellor at this time.

Researchers have found that an abortion does not generally make a woman feel bad about herself years later.

Do many teenagers have abortions?
About 45% of pregnant teenagers choose to have an abortion.

Unfortunately, many other teenagers decide to have an abortion too late in their pregnancies. Either they don't realise they are pregnant or they don't know what to do about it.

That is why it is important to see someone if you think you are pregnant as then you can get all the help you need and as quickly as possible.

Is it wrong to have an abortion?
Some religions think that abortion is wrong. For example Roman Catholics. This is because they believe that life begins at the moment of conception and should be protected from this time.

However, other people believe that abortion is a responsible decision, when a woman cannot handle a pregnancy or is in the situation to take care of a child properly.

It all comes down to everybody's personal beliefs and opinions.

Is it legal to have an abortion?
It is in most countries. For example, it is legal in England, Wales and Scotland but not in Northern Ireland or the Irish Republic where abortion is illegal. This is because the Irish religion is Roman Catholic.

What happens if I live in Ireland?
This is a very difficult question to answer. By law, Irish women must follow the law and respect their religion that abortion is illegal in their country. However, as time has moved on, people realise that we are all beginning to follow personally chosen religion and beliefs.

Marie Stopes International can still help if you do have an unplanned pregnancy and live in Ireland. There is a centre based in Dublin which can help you with advice and counselling. If you did choose to go ahead with an abortion, you would then have to travel to England for the procedure.

■ The above information is from Pupiline's web site which can be found at www.pupiline.net

Teenage pregnancy

If your period is late and you think you might be pregnant take the following steps . . .

Do a pregnancy test

They are FREE at Brook Centres, some GPs, many family planning clinics and at some GUM clinics . . . the testing is confidential and only you and the nurse will know what's going on.

Hate the idea of talking to someone? For about £10 you can buy a home pregnancy test – all you do is go to your local pharmacy or supermarket where they sell a range of reliable testing kits. Follow the instructions carefully though if you want a reliable result.

The result will either be:

Negative – if you don't want to be pregnant you will breathe a sigh of relief and use this false alarm to get your contraception sorted out! See your GP, family planning clinic or use condoms.

Positive – you now need to decide what to do. Other people/doctors/counsellors can help you make a decision by explaining your choices but in the end you must decide what you want.

Your choices:
- keep the baby
- adoption
- abortion

Who can you talk to?

If you are pregnant, and the pregnancy is unplanned you may be feeling confused, shocked, and scared but try not to let this stop you from seeking help. It is important to face what is happening and seek advice as soon as possible, so all options are open to you and you can begin your maternity care.

It is also important to make the right decision for you, and this might not always be the decision your boyfriend or your parents would make. Try and talk it over with someone you trust.

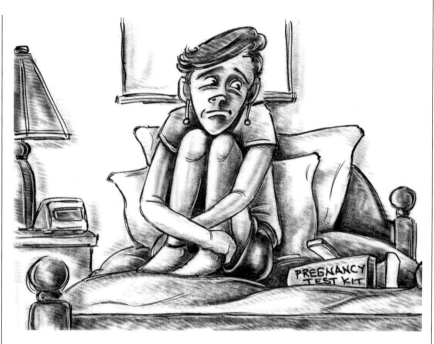

Talking it over

You could talk it over with your boyfriend or your mum or dad, but if you don't feel you can talk to them, you could also speak to: an older sister or brother, your friends, a teacher, a doctor, a social worker, a school counsellor, your GP, Brook Advisory Counsellor, or Marie Stopes International (MSI) counsellor.

Whoever you talk to it's important to seek help from organisations that are impartial. For example, anti-abortion organisations will not provide unbiased or objective information.

How does pregnancy happen?

Pregnancy (conception) occurs when a sperm fertilises an egg by joining with it during sex. This can happen when two people have sex and do not use contraception.

A fertilised egg will then move down into a girl's uterus and implant itself into the womb (uterus) lining where it will begin to grow.

Are you old enough to do it?

If you're old enough to do 'it' you're old enough to be responsible for what can happen.

Whether you're male or female, with the decision to have sex, comes the responsibility of being sensible and protecting yourself from an unplanned pregnancy.

This basically means understanding how pregnancy happens and how you can stop it.

If you've got an appointment to have a pregnancy test at a clinic – don't forget . . .

The date of the first day of your last period.

Some of your first wee that morning – in a clean jar with a tight fitting lid.

Most clinics offer a pregnancy testing service for free – but check before you go.

If you're doing the test yourself remember to follow the instructions carefully – if you don't it could effect the results!

Keeping the baby

What happens if I decide to keep the baby?

First, see a GP who will organise maternity care for you, tell you what to expect, what you should be eating and what check-ups you need to go for.

If you are bringing up the baby on your own and need somewhere to live, you need to contact social services (your GP may be able to do this for you). Social services will be able to give you advice about benefits that you may be entitled to.

Specific organisations exist to help single parents.

Having the baby adopted
What happens if I put the baby up for adoption?
First, contact your local social services department (your GP will be able to help you).

You cannot arrange the adoption yourself unless your child is to be adopted by a close relative.

When does the adoption process begin?
Social services will work with approved adoption agencies to arrange preparation for adoption before your child is born, but nothing will be definitely arranged until after the birth. You will be completely free to change your mind.

The social worker will discuss with you the kind of family you want your child to grow up in and will usually tell you quite a lot about the family that is likely to become the baby's new parents.

You should talk to the social worker about the possibility of meeting the family, if you want to, or about other sorts of contact you could have in the future.

When does the adoption process become legal?
Although social workers arrange adoptions, they are made legally binding by the courts.

The court will make sure that you are definite about your decision to put your baby up for adoption and that the baby's new home is the right environment for him/her to grow up in.

The adoption is usually made legal three months after the birth of the child.

What if I change my mind?
Everyone recognises that putting a child up for adoption is a very big step for a mother so you have at least six weeks after the birth before you need to give your final agreement in writing to the court.

When the adoption order has been agreed by the court you will no longer have any legal relationship with or responsibilities for your child.

Is adoption the same as fostering?
No, adoption means legally giving up responsibility for your child. Fostering means that another set of parents will temporarily look after your baby but that you will remain the legal guardian and hopefully be in a position to care for your child in the future.

The same people who organise adoption can help you with fostering. If, for whatever reason, you cannot look after your baby, social services will arrange temporary fostering and will try to work with you to reunite you with your child. Making a decision about adoption or fostering is a big one and you should feel able to take time to make the right decision for you and speak to organisations and people who can help you make up your mind.

For more help and advice on adoption contact: The British Agencies for Adoption and Fostering (BAAF), 11 Southwark Street, London SE1 1RQ. Tel: 0207 593 2000.

Abortion: ending the pregnancy
What happens if I decide to have an abortion?
Firstly, see your GP, MSI or Brook for information about the type of abortion available to you.

You could also ask to see a counsellor at the clinic as they will go through the feelings you may have before and after.

Their aim is to help you cope with what you are going through and help you make the right decision. Both the doctor and the counsellor will discuss if you want your parents to know about your abortion.

While you can give consent (agree to an abortion) under 16, a doctor will only give the go-ahead if

---

Remember, you have choices so make sure that all options are clearly explained to you

---

s/he believes you understand what's involved.

Even if a doctor agrees, they may still encourage you to involve a parent (though they will not go behind your back and tell your parents).

Who can I take with me?
Lots of women prefer to go with someone to support them. You can take anyone, from a friend, a relative, or a parent to a boyfriend or a brother or sister.

Abortion options:
What kinds of abortion are there?
What kind of abortion you have very much depends on:
- how many weeks pregnant you are
- whether or not you want a general anaesthetic (without one you will be awake during the procedure)
- whether or not you are suitable for a medical abortion (you will be given pills to end your pregnancy).

The earlier you go for help the more options are available so don't put off seeking advice.

Remember, you have choices so make sure that all options are clearly explained to you by the nurse/doctor and don't be afraid to ask questions.

What happens afterwards?
After you have ended your pregnancy you will probably feel cramps very like your period cramps, and experience some bleeding which can last up to 14 days.

The nurses will tell you what to expect, and how to look after yourself. They will also make you a follow-up appointment to make sure there are no problems.

Finally, a doctor will also discuss having sex again. While this may be the last thing on your mind, you need to know how long to wait after your abortion and what contraception to use. If you want to talk to someone after your abortion most hospitals and organisations like MSI offer post-abortion counselling.

■ The above information is from Marie Stopes International's web site www.likeitis.org.uk

Abortions carried out on under-16s soar

By Steve Doughty

The number of abortions on under-age girls has risen by around a quarter over the last decade despite Government efforts to cut teenage pregnancies.

There were 4,382 terminations on under-16s in 2000 compared with 3,510 in 1992, according to figures obtained by MPs from the Office for National Statistics.

The new total includes 234 abortions on girls under 14.

Britain has the highest teenage pregnancy rate in Europe and, since 1992, the number of abortions among under-16s has risen relentlessly. Occasional falls have proved to be temporary blips.

The figure for 2000 was an increase of 200 on the previous year.

Yet the year 2000 saw the introduction of a programme in which teenagers were freely offered the morning-after pill.

It began with a trial in Manchester which was said to have 'prevented' 700 pregnancies in six months. By the end of the year, the pill could be bought over the counter at chemists for £10.

However, the latest figures show that the introduction of the national policy did nothing to cut under-age pregnancy and abortion in its first phase.

The number of pregnancies among under-16s in 2000 went up by 161 to 8,111 – the first rise in five years.

According to figures for England and Wales alone there were just over 3,800 abortions on girls under 16 in 2000.

> ## There were 4,382 terminations on under-16s in 2000 compared with 3,510 in 1992

In 1997, the year Labour came to power, there were 3,400.

The figures add to the growing evidence that Government-backed efforts to cut teenage pregnancy by giving all schoolgirls sex education and easy access to contraception and the morning-after pill are failing.

On Saturday, the *Daily Mail* reported that some Tesco stores are handing out free morning-after pills to teenagers in a pilot project aimed at halving pregnancy rates.

Nuala Scarisbrick, of the anti-abortion charity Life, said: 'The Government think the morning-after pill is a cure for everything.

'But the strategy is not working to cut numbers of pregnancies.

'It is also leaving girls exposed to the risks of sexually-transmitted diseases, which are already at epidemic levels.

'For young girls, the consequences can be very serious – for example chlamydia can cause infertility.'

There is a growing debate over long-established official views that young girls become pregnant because they are ignorant about sex or cannot obtain contraceptives.

Research carried out at Nottingham University, and published this month, suggests that providing contraception and advice either makes no difference to pregnancy rates or makes them worse.

The official policy fails to work because, although it means sexually-active teenagers are less likely to fall pregnant, it encourages many more teenagers to have sex.

Ministers, however, have been claiming success for their policy on the basis of small falls in pregnancy rates among girls aged between 16 and 18.

© The Daily Mail, 2003

Teenage conception rates

England and Wales — Rates per 1,000 conceptions

	Leading to maternities					Leading to abortion				
	1971	1981	1991	1996	1999	1971	1981	1991	1996	1999
Age at conception										
Under 14[1]	0.5	0.4	0.5	0.6	0.5	0.5	0.7	0.7	0.8	0.7
14	2.8	1.7	2.6	2.7	2.4	2.4	2.9	3.5	3.6	3.3
15	13.5	7.1	9.8	11.0	9.0	6.9	8.7	9.3	9.4	9.2
All aged under 16[1]	5.5	3.1	4.3	4.8	3.9	3.2	4.1	4.6	4.7	4.4
16	41.0	21.5	25.0	27.1	24.0	13.0	16.2	17.1	17.9	18.8
17	68.5	36.7	41.5	42.5	40.8	15.2	20.1	22.7	24.1	25.9
18	95.0	54.6	57.0	56.5	53.5	16.7	21.6	26.6	29.2	30.3
19	114.5	73.0	66.2	66.5	61.6	16.4	21.0	28.6	31.4	32.4
All aged under 20[1]	67.3	38.9	42.0	40.4	38.6	14.3	18.2	22.1	23.0	24.3

1 Rates for girls aged under 14, under 16 and under 20 are based on the population of girls aged 13, 13 to 15 and 15 to 19, respectively.

Source: Office for National Statistics, Crown copyright

Unwanted pregnancy and abortion

Some questions answered

Could I be pregnant?

If you have had sex without using a contraceptive or the contraceptive you use has failed, you could be pregnant.

Emergency contraception can prevent an unwanted pregnancy if the woman is treated within 72 hours of unprotected sex, but the sooner it is used the more likely it is to work. Pills are available from some doctors, family planning clinics or Brook Advisory Centres, or you could have an IUD (intra-uterine device) fitted.

What are the symptoms of pregnancy?

The most common sign of possible pregnancy is a missed period. Other signs are sickness, swollen breasts and passing urine more frequently

What do I do if I miss my period?

If your period is a week overdue you should go for a pregnancy test. Your doctor should be able to do this. However, if you do not want to go to your doctor, go to your local Family Planning Clinic, Brook Advisory Centre, or buy a home-test kit from a chemist. It is important that you seek help as early as possible because

if you decide you do not want to continue the pregnancy and you want to seek an abortion, the earlier it is done in the pregnancy the safer it is for you.

If your pregnancy test is negative but you miss another period you should have a repeat test.

If I am pregnant, what can I do?

There are three options open to you.

Firstly, if your pregnancy is unplanned, you may decide to continue with it and have a child. If this is the case, you should go to your doctor and arrange ante-natal care.

Secondly, you may decide to continue with the pregnancy and have the child adopted. Details of adoption agencies may be obtained from Citizens' Advice Bureaux, social services at your local council, local churches, the Family Planning Association, etc.

Thirdly, you may decide to seek an abortion.

Who can I talk to?

Whatever your final decision you may want to discuss all the options

with someone else. This could be your doctor or a counsellor at a Family Planning Clinic or the Brook Advisory Centre. If you feel you can, you should discuss it with your parents, although you may be nervous of their reaction.

If you are under sixteen years of age and wish to seek an abortion your parents will normally need to be involved in the decision. If, however, you have strong reasons for not wanting them to know, your doctor is legally able to agree to the abortion without your parents' knowledge or consent so long as you show that you fully understand what it means to have an abortion.

What is an abortion?

An abortion is when a pregnancy is ended before a baby is capable of surviving on its own outside the mother's body. An abortion can either happen naturally, i.e. a miscarriage, or it can be induced, i.e. done deliberately. An induced abortion is only legal if it is carried out within the law and in the circumstances which the law permits.

NEVER attempt to induce an abortion yourself as this could cause you serious injury.

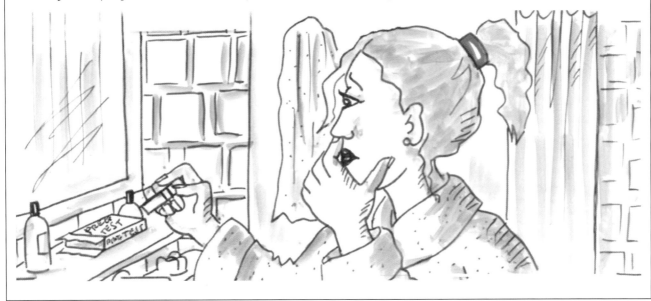

What does the law say about abortion?

Under the terms of the Abortion Act, a woman requires the agreement of two doctors before an abortion may be carried out. Doctors can agree to an abortion if they believe one or more of the following:

a. continuing with the pregnancy would involve more risk to your physical or mental health than terminating it.

b. continuing with the pregnancy would involve greater risk to your life than terminating it.

c. any existing children of yours would be likely to suffer if the pregnancy continued.

d. there is a substantial risk that the child would be seriously disabled.

A doctor can take into account your financial and social circumstances when considering your request for an abortion, if you are less than 24 weeks pregnant.

Where should I go if I decide to seek an abortion?

You should first go to your doctor. If the doctor agrees to your request you would normally be referred to a local NHS hospital and seen by another doctor, who, if agreeable to the abortion, would make the arrangements for your admission to hospital.

In some cases (partly depending on where you live) NHS facilities may not be available for abortion and you may be referred to either a non-profit making clinic dealing with abortion or a private clinic. In these circumstances you may have to pay for the abortion.

What do I do if the doctor will not help me?

Some doctors do not agree with abortion, although they should refer

---

If you are having sex and do not want a child, it is essential that you seek contraceptive advice and choose a method of contraception that suits you

---

you to another doctor. Other women for personal reasons may not wish to go to their doctor. In these circumstances you should go for help to one of the following: Family Planning Association, a Brook Advisory Centre, the British Pregnancy Advisory Service, Marie Stopes International, or a Citizens' Advice Bureau.

What does abortion involve?

In the first nine weeks of pregnancy you may be able to take pills to bring on an abortion or in the first three months you could have a surgical operation which is a very simple procedure carried out under either local or general anaesthetic. If the abortion is carried out in a day care unit you could be out of hospital or clinic on the same day. In other places you may have to stay overnight. If you are later into the pregnancy, the simpler abortion techniques may not be possible and you will have to stay in hospital a little longer.

How can I reduce the risks of an unwanted pregnancy?

If you are having sex and do not want a child, it is essential that you seek contraceptive advice and choose a method of contraception that suits you.

If you do not want to go to your own doctor, use your local Family Planning Clinic or Brook Advisory Centre. (Brook Advisory Centres give particular help to under-25-year-olds.)

Remember: If the contraceptive you use fails (i.e. a burst condom) or you forget to use your contraceptive, emergency contraception used within 72 hours of unprotected sex can prevent an unwanted pregnancy.

One of the following organisations will be able to refer you to somewhere near you where you can get help:

Brook Advisory Centres (for under 25-year-olds)
165 Grays Inn Road, London WC1X 8UD. Tel: 0800 0185023

Family Planning Association
2-12 Pentonville Road, London N1 9FP. Tel: 020 7837 4044

British Pregnancy Advisory Service*
Austy Manor, Wootton Wawen, Solihull, West Midlands B95 6BX. Tel: 08457 304030

Marie Stopes International*
108 Whitfield Street, London W1P 6BE. Tel: 0845 300 8090

Citizens' Advice Bureau
(Address and telephone number in telephone directory.)
* Provide emergency contraception for a fee.

■ The above information is from the Abortion Law Reform Association's web site which can be found at www.alra.org.uk

© *The Abortion Law Reform Association (ALRA)*

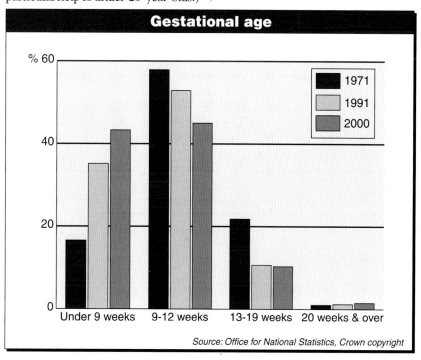
Gestational age

Source: Office for National Statistics, Crown copyright

Abortion and religion

Information from Education for Choice

Over a third of all pregnancies, across the world, are unplanned.[1] The discovery of an unplanned pregnancy affects all women differently. Each woman's circumstances are unique and there are sometimes reasons why she may not feel able to continue with a pregnancy.

Although some religions oppose abortion under all circumstances, many religions recognise the different factors that influence a woman's decision on how to proceed with a pregnancy and teach that there are *some* instances in which abortion is acceptable. Most religions agree that abortion is a last resort; they teach that the decision to have an abortion is a serious one and must not be taken lightly.

This article looks at some of the key moral questions that influence religious thought on abortion as well as looking at the teachings of some of the major world religions.

What are the key questions for people of different faiths?

When does life begin?

Not all religions define a particular moment when life begins but some, like Buddhism, Sikhism and Catholicism, teach that life begins at fertilisation – the moment that sperm meets egg. The Roman Catholic Church says that the fertilised egg is a sacred life, with as many rights as a baby, child or adult, and forbids abortion. Amongst Buddhists and Sikhs there is a variety of opinions on the morality of abortion.

Medical science tells us that a proportion of fertilised eggs do not become implanted in the woman's womb and that a large proportion of those that do (up to 25%) are lost naturally to miscarriage. This loss of 'life' is often not acknowledged in any formalised religious ritual – such as a funeral – and in many cases the woman might not even know that she was pregnant or that she has miscarried.

Who has the greater right to life: the fetus or the woman?

The Roman Catholic Church says that abortion – 'the deliberate ending of a pregnancy' – is never acceptable, even to save the life of the woman. However, life-saving treatment can be carried out on a woman even if it will result in the death of the fetus. So, in this particular situation, the woman does have a greater right to life than the fetus.[2]

Most religions would choose to save the life of the woman even at the cost of the fetus. Even religions that are firmly opposed to abortion like the Greek and Russian Orthodox Churches, Hinduism and Orthodox Judaism say that abortion is acceptable to save a woman's life.

Some religions go further than this and teach that the woman has the right to decide on the fate of the fetus even if continuing with the pregnancy does not directly threaten her life. It is argued by some Christians that God has given human beings free will and that we must respect the integrity of woman's conscience. To remove her choice is to deny that integrity and, in effect, her humanity.

Is abortion murder?

Most religions teach about the sanctity or sacredness of human life, but do not categorise abortion as murder.

Judaism, for example, only recognises the rights of a baby after the majority of the baby has left the woman's body, so although it teaches that abortion is morally wrong, it is not considered equivalent to murder.

Despite the general prohibition on killing – for example Judaism and Christianity teach 'Thou Shalt Not Kill' (Exodus and Deuteronomy) whilst Muslims believe ' . . . whosoever kills a human being . . . it shall be as if he had killed all mankind' (Quran 5:32) – most religions recognise that not all killing is murder. Killing in battle, in self-defence, as legal punishment or retribution is sanctioned by many religions.

Does the fetus have a soul?

Islam teaches that ensoulment (the moment that the soul enters the body of the fetus) takes place at 120 days and abortions after this time are considered to be more of a sin than early abortions.

The Roman Catholic Church used to teach that ensoulment takes place at 'quickening' when the woman starts to feel movement in her stomach (about 16 weeks).

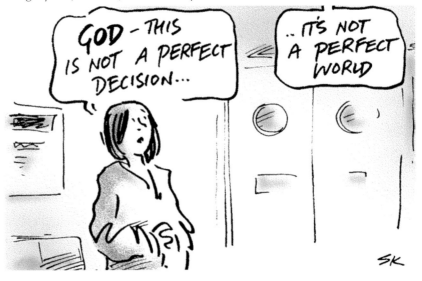

However in 1869 the church changed its teaching and it now teaches that the soul is present from the moment of fertilisation.

Hindus believe that the fetus has a soul, although opinion is divided over what happens to the soul of an aborted fetus. Some believe that the soul, like all souls of the dead, will be reincarnated in another body.

Quakers believe that there is 'that of God in everyone' but do not give guidance on whether this applies to the fetus.

When does a fetus become a person?

This question is important because we do not give human rights (such as the right to life) to all living things (plants, animals etc.) but only to people.

The earliest embryo contains the entire DNA code (genome) of the person that could develop from it, and some argue that its potential to become a person is enough to give it the rights of a fully developed person.

Others argue that a person is more than just the sum of its biological parts, and believe that a living person has characteristics that a fetus doesn't. These may include the ability to think and reason or the capacity to build relationships and to communicate.

Some believe that it is the ability of the fetus to exist independently of the woman that defines it as a person. They consider the fetus to have the right to life at the point where it is 'viable', meaning it can survive outside of the woman's womb. (British law recognises viability as an important indicator of person-hood and gives greater rights to the fetus after this point in its development.)

Most religions agree that gesta-tion (the fetus growing in the womb) is a process of becoming a person and consequently teach that later abor-tions are morally worse than early abortions.

Religion, the law and practice

There is not always a connection between a country's main religion and its abortion laws.

Where do world religions stand on abortion?

Some religions, notably the monotheistic faiths, rely on one or two key texts and have clear doctrine on moral issues. Others, such as Hinduism and Buddhism, consist of collections of writings which are more open to interpretation. Some religions like Islam have maintained a relatively consistent teaching on abortion while others, like Roman Catholicism, have changed their ideas on abortion over time. The information below aims to give a broad overview of the teaching of different religions on abortion.[3]

Prohibited
The Roman Catholic Church teaches that abortion is always wrong. A Catholic who had an abortion could, in theory, be 'excommunicated' from the church.
The Jehovah's Witnesses believe that abortion is always wrong.
The Evangelical Christian movement includes many who are totally opposed to all abortion.

Very restricted
The Russian and Greek Orthodox Churches teach that abortion can only be justified to save a woman's life.
Orthodox Judaism believes that abortion can only be justified to save the woman's life or to protect her from the risk of serious and permanent injury.
Hinduism is opposed to abortion, but some Hindu texts approve of abortion to save a woman's life.

Limited
The Church of England considers that abortion is sometimes a 'necessary evil'. Later abortions are worse than early abortions.
Islam teaches that abortion is a sin which increases as the pregnancy progresses, but does allow for its use to save the life or protect the health of the woman and in other limited circumstances.
Liberal/Reform Judaism leaves the decision to the woman and her partner, but is clear that abortion should not be used for 'trivial reasons'.

No written law
Buddhism
Some say that abortions break the first rule of Buddhism, which is to 'do no harm'. Others believe in compassion for the individual woman in this situation.

Sikhism
Decisions on contraception are left entirely up to the married couple to decide and some also believe that abortion too is possible if both partners agree. Others say that it is forbidden.

Quakers
There is no official teaching on abortion. However, there is a great emphasis on personal conscience and the individual's capacity to make good decisions.

Individual decision
Humanists believe that the quality rather than quantity of life is important and that there is nothing wrong in principle with abortion. Rational thought should direct our actions, so women should have the opportunity to weigh up the pros and cons of abortion and make their own decisions.

The Methodist Church spoke out to highlight the dangers of illegal abortions before the law was changed in 1967. It teaches that you should have reverence for life and also have compassion for women who are not able to continue with a pregnancy.

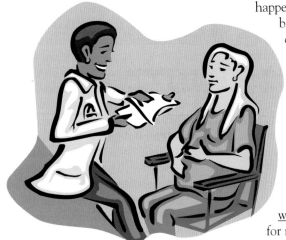

Most Latin American countries prohibit or severely restrict abortion which is in keeping with Roman Catholic teaching.

India, which has a majority Hindu population, has very liberal abortion laws that do not reflect mainstream Hindu teaching on abortion.

Egypt and Iran completely prohibit abortion despite the exception that Islam makes to preserve women's life or health.

The official teaching of a religion is not always reflected in the way its members actually live their lives. Many people feel that they must make decisions based on their own conscience and circumstances, even when they do not fit in with the official teachings of their religion or their own faith. Abortion is a good example of this as it takes place in every culture and every country in the world often in opposition to the community's culture, religion or law. Statistics show that people of all religions have abortions and that the numbers of abortions that take place do not relate to the law or religion of the country.

Four million abortions a year take place in Latin America and 6,000 Irish women travel to Britain each year for abortions because it is prohibited in those countries by law and religion. 26% of the world's population live in countries where abortion is prohibited, but many of those countries have a high abortion rate. An estimated 70,000 women die each year through illegal abortions, demonstrating that prohibiting abortion does not prevent it from happening, but makes it unsafe by removing access to doctors and sanitary medical facilities.[4]

Notes

1 According to the Safe Motherhood Initiative, 75 million of the 200 million pregnancies that take place around the world each year are unplanned. See www.safemotherhood.org for more information.

2 For example, a life-threatening ectopic pregnancy (in which the fertilised egg is implanted in the fallopian tube instead of the womb) can be ended, by removing the whole fallopian tube, but not the fertilised egg on its own because according to Catholic law it must be the 'damaged' organ not the fetus that is being intentionally removed. (*Abortion*, Catholic Truth Society www.cts-online.org.uk).

3 For more detailed information and quotes from different religions visit our website at www.efc.org.uk

4 World Health Organisation.

■ The above information is from Education for Choice's web site which can be found at www.efc.org.uk

© Education for Choice

LIFE says attitudes to abortion are changing

LIFE, the UK's leading prolife charity, welcomes the report in the *Daily Mail* today, which predicts that a sea-change in attitudes to abortion taking place in the US is crossing over to the UK.

Speaking today, LIFE Trustee Nuala Scarisbrick said: 'It has always been our hope that people in the UK would gradually realise that for years they have been conned by pro-abortion propaganda. The truth is now coming out and prolife values are beginning to prevail over the so-called "pro-choice" lobby.

'Everyone, from the medical establishment to ordinary men and women, is beginning to see that the abortionism of the last 35 years has been a terrible mistake. Millions of babies have lost their lives and millions of women have undergone a horrible experience. Many men, too, have been denied the chance to raise their children.

'The link between abortion and breast cancer is accepted in more and more quarters of the medical profession in the face of irrefutable evidence. Increasing numbers of women are succumbing to breast cancer who have undergone previous abortions. Many women's fertility has been damaged as they find they cannot have children because of a previous abortion, and countless women have suffered the traumatic psychological after-effects of abortion known as post-abortion syndrome (PAS).

'But perhaps most tellingly, in the UK, as in America, it is those women who have undergone abortion themselves that are most fervently against it. Many who have been traumatised by the experience want to prevent other women suffering in the same way. They are beginning to sue abortion doctors because they were not warned of the havoc which abortion can do to minds and bodies. The first cases in the UK are under way.

'We hope that this change in attitudes leads to the provision of first-class pregnancy care for women and proper support for families in the UK. Only then will abortion become unnecessary and women will have real choice and freedom.'

■ The above information is from LIFE's web site which can be found at www.lifeuk.org

© LIFE 2003

A non-religious perspective on abortion

On moral questions, humanists are guided by principles based on reason and respect for others, not obedience to dogmatic rules. Abortion is a subject that demonstrates the difficulties of rigid rules in moral decision making. Medical science has advanced to the point where we have options that were unthinkable even a few generations ago and where old rules cannot cope with new facts.

Some medical facts

Some very premature babies can now be kept alive, which has altered ideas about when foetuses become human beings with human rights.

Many illnesses and disabilities can now be diagnosed long before birth.

- Some very ill or disabled babies who would probably once have died before or shortly after birth can now be kept alive.
- The sex of a foetus can be known well before birth (and some parents would like to be able to choose the sex of their child).
- Genetic research makes it increasingly likely that parents will be able to know, or even to choose, other characteristics for their unborn child. A few will want to reject some foetuses.
- Abortions can be performed safely, though they can occasionally cause medical or psychological problems.

These are in themselves morally neutral medical facts, but they bring with them the necessity to make moral choices and to consider who should make those choices. Doctors? Politicians? Religious leaders? Medical ethics committees? Individual women? Their partners?

Some views on abortion

Some examples of contemporary rules and views about abortion will perhaps demonstrate the complexity of the problem:

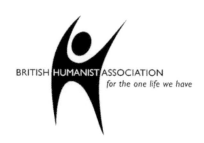

- Some religious people think that all human life is sacred, that life begins at conception, and so abortion is always wrong (and some also believe that contraception is wrong, which leads to even more unwanted pregnancies). But if one has to choose between risking the life of the mother or the life of the unborn foetus, how does one decide

---

Abortion is a subject that demonstrates the difficulties of rigid rules in moral decision making

---

whose life is more 'sacred'? (This is very rare these days, and the choice is most often about the quality of life of either the mother or the foetus or both.)

- People often argue that it is not for doctors 'to play God' and that it is for God to decide matters of life and death. But it could be said that all medical interventions are 'playing God' (even your childhood vaccinations may have kept you alive longer than 'God' planned) so we have to decide for ourselves how we use medical powers. Arguments which invoke God are unconvincing to those who do not believe in gods, and laws should not be based on claims which rely on religious faith.
- Some moral philosophers have argued that full consciousness begins only after birth or even later, and so foetuses and infants are not full human beings with human rights.
- Doctors have a range of opinions on abortion, but tend to give the medical interests of the mother (which may include her mental health) the most weight when making decisions.

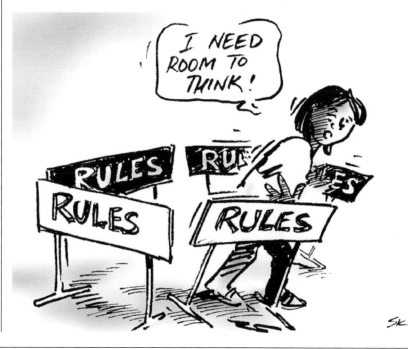

- Some doctors and nurses dislike carrying out abortions because they feel that their job is to save life, not to destroy it.
- Some people believe that a woman has absolute rights over her own body which override those of any unborn foetus. You might like to read Judith Jarvis Thomson's *A Defense of Abortion* which states a feminist case for abortion very clearly.
- The law in England, Scotland and Wales is based on the fact that after twenty-four weeks the foetus is often viable, in that with medical care it can survive outside the womb.
- The law in England, Scotland and Wales states that an abortion can be performed before the twenty-fourth week of pregnancy if two doctors agree that there is a risk to the life or the mental or physical health of the mother if the pregnancy continues, or there will be a risk to the mental or physical health of other children in the family. However, there is no time limit if there is a substantial risk that the baby will be born severely disabled, or there is a grave risk of death or permanent injury (mental or physical) to the mother. In effect this means that almost every woman who wants an abortion and is persistent in seeking one before the twenty-fourth week can obtain one. However, some women who do not realise that they are pregnant till too late (perhaps because they are very young or because they are menopausal) may not be able to have abortions though they would have qualified on other grounds.

The humanist view

So how do humanists pick their way between these conflicting ideas? Humanists respect life and value happiness and personal choice, so they might agree with many of the above points. And in a democratic nation such as the UK, they would respect and obey the law, though they recognise that the law is not always the same as justice or morality, and would campaign for changes when they consider laws to be unjust. In any case, the current law is simply permissive; it does not impose abortion on anyone who does not want it, so even within the law, people have to make moral choices.

Because humanists take happiness and suffering into consideration, they are more concerned with the quality of life than the right to life, if the two come into conflict. The probable quality of life of the baby, the woman, the father and the rest of the family, the doctors and nurses involved, would all have to be given due weight. There is plenty of room for debate about how much weight each individual should have, but most humanists would probably put the interests of the woman first, since she would have to complete the pregnancy and probably care for the baby, whose happiness would largely depend on hers. She also exists already with other responsibilities and rights and desires which can be taken into account – unlike those of the unborn foetus which cannot be so surely ascertained.

Of course all possible options should be explored and decisions should be informed ones. Adoption of the unwanted baby might be a better solution in some cases. On reflection a woman might decide that she could look after a sick or disabled child. Or she might decide that she cannot offer this child a life worth living and abortion is the better choice. She will need to consider the long-term effects as well as the immediate ones. It is unlikely to be an easy decision, and requiring an abortion is a situation that most women would prefer to avoid.

For society as a whole, as well as for the children themselves, it is better if every child is a wanted child. However, abortion is not the best way of avoiding unwanted children, and improved sex education, easily available contraception, and better education and opportunities for young women, can all help to reduce the number of abortions. But as long as abortion is needed as a last resort, most humanists would agree that society should provide safe legal facilities. The alternatives, which would inevitably include illegal abortions, are far worse.

Questions to think about

- Is abortion in the case of conception after rape more justified than other abortions?
- Would a humanist favour abortion if a woman wanted one because her pregnancy was interfering with her holiday plans? Why (not)?
- Why do humanists think contraception is better than abortion?
- Are there any good arguments against adoption of unwanted babies?
- Should doctors and nurses impose their moral views on patients? Yes? Sometimes? Never?
- Should religious people impose their views on abortion on non-religious people? Yes? Sometimes? Never?
- Should parents be able to choose the sex of their child? Should they be able to abort a foetus of the 'wrong' sex?
- At what point does a foetus become a human being? Does it make any difference to the humanist view of abortion?
- Can infanticide ever be right?
- Should abortion ever be carried out on a non-consenting woman, e.g. one too young to give legal consent or one in a coma?
- How are you deciding your answers to these questions?

- The above information is from the British Humanist Association's web site which can be found at www.humanism.org.uk

© British Humanist Association (BHA)

Abortion and the law

Information from Brook Advisory Centres

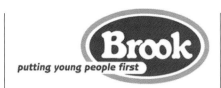

Two Acts of Parliament, the Abortion Act 1967 and the Human Fertilisation and Embryology Act 1990, regulate the provision of abortion in England, Wales and Scotland.

The Abortion Act requires that two doctors must agree to an abortion and that it must be carried out by a registered practitioner in an NHS hospital or a location that has been approved by the Department of Health. The Abortion Act gives medical staff the legal right not to participate in abortions if they have a moral objection to the treatment. Section 37 of the Human Fertilisation and Embryology Act governs the time limits for abortion. Taken together, the two Acts provide that abortion is legal on the following grounds:

a. the continuance of the pregnancy would involve risk to the life of the pregnant woman greater than if the pregnancy were terminated.

b. the termination is necessary to prevent grave permanent injury to the physical or mental health of the pregnant woman.

c. the pregnancy has not exceeded 24 weeks and the continuance of the pregnancy would involve risk, greater than if the pregnancy were terminated, of injury to the physical or mental health of the pregnant woman.

d. the pregnancy has not exceeded 24 weeks and the continuance of the pregnancy would involve risk, greater than if the pregnancy were terminated, of injury to the physical or mental health of any existing child(ren) of the family of the pregnant woman.

e. there is a substantial risk that if the child were born it would suffer from such physical or mental abnormalities as to be seriously handicapped.

There is no time limit on grounds a), b) and e). The Abortion Act and Section 37 of the Human Fertilisation and Embryology Act do not apply to Northern Ireland.

In Jersey, the legal framework is set by the Termination of Pregnancy (Jersey) Law 1997 which allows for abortion if two doctors agree that one of the following applies:

■ the woman is no more than 12 weeks pregnant and her condition causes her distress.

■ the woman is no more than 24 weeks pregnant and the foetus is suffering from a severe incurable abnormality which would cause it to be born with the expectation of an exceedingly poor quality of life.

■ a termination is necessary to save the woman's life or to prevent grave permanent injury to her physical or mental health.

Doctors who have a strong moral objection to abortion are not required to be involved. However, the British Medical Association and the Department of Health have ruled that such doctors should make arrangements for their patients to see another doctor who is willing to advise about abortion.

If a young woman under 16 is considered competent to consent to her own medical treatment, she can consent to an abortion. However, it is usually only in extreme situations that an abortion would be performed without any parental involvement.

A potential father has no legal rights over a foetus. The decision to terminate a pregnancy is made between the woman and her doctor.

■ The above information is from Brook Advisory Centres' web site which can be found at www.brook.org.uk

© Brook Advisory Centres

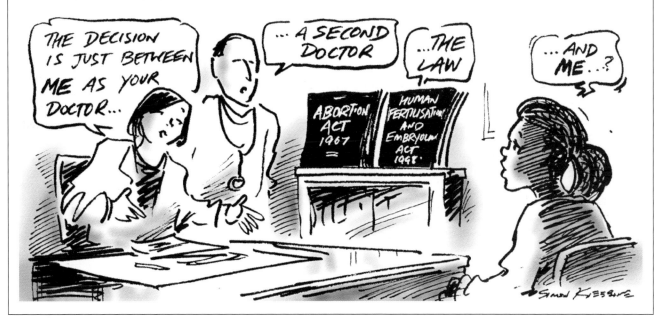

Pro-life or pro-choice?

Information from Pupiline

People often have very strong views about abortion. As I keep stating, it will always come down to the individual and their religion, upbringing, experiences and beliefs which will explain their personal view on abortion. To make us all a bit wiser and to understand everyone's view on abortion, here are the arguments for and against abortion. Read this to be clued up on everyone's right of opinion and beliefs:

Pro-life

People are often against legal abortion because they believe that:

- Human life begins at conception and abortion destroys respect for human life
- Abortion is a violent act that damages a mother and her baby. It is uncivilised and unjust
- There are alternatives to abortion, such as adoption
- Abortion damages women because they suffer post-abortion guilt and trauma
- Abortion is rarely necessary to safe the life of the woman
- Abortion encourages brutality and child-abuse
- Abortion on grounds of foetal abnormality encourages discrimination against disabled people

Pro-choice

People are often for legal abortion because they believe that:

- The embryo or foetus should be respected as potential human life but does not have the same value as a born person
- Women are capable of making the right moral choices and can follow their own consciences

People often have very strong views about abortion, it will always come down to the individual and their religion, upbringing, experiences and beliefs

- A pregnant woman understands her own personal circumstances better than anyone else and so is in the best position to know whether she should or should not have a child
- Legal abortion is relatively safe and is likely to cause the woman less harm than forcing her to continue her pregnancy and have an unwanted child
- It is better for children to be born to parents who want them and love them
- Public opinion supports legal abortion
- When abortion is illegal women tend to travel elsewhere because they are so desperate to avoid having to continue an unwanted pregnancy

Whatever your opinion, there is help out there for those who are pregnant and in need of help – even if it is just advice you want.

It is nice to have the freedom of choice. But it is always important to respect other people's opinions – whether you are pro-choice or pro-life, respect everyone else's view as well!

- The above information is from Pupiline's web site which can be found at www.pupiline.net

© 1999-2003 Pupiline Limited

Hard questions answered

Information from LIFE

Backstreet abortions?
This term is usually used for illegal abortions which are not performed in hospitals or clinics.

Even before the 1967 Abortion Act, the number of women in danger after backstreet abortions was getting smaller. It is, of course, impossible to produce accurate figures for such illegal activities, but the numbers of women admitted to hospital after botched abortions was on the way

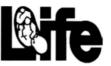

down years before 1967. Many so-called 'backstreet 'abortions before 1967 were done in 'front' streets, e.g. Harley Street and similar, i.e. by private practice gynaecologists. Backstreet abortions were almost always performed early in pregnancy

The development of the child makes later abortions difficult to perform without medical facilities.

Those who think abortion is wrong reject backstreet abortions along with all other abortions. It is not where, or how badly, they are performed, that makes the difference. Wherever or however they are performed, at least one life is ended, sometimes two. And to argue that we must legalise abortion because there will always be an illegal backstreet trade is like saying that we must legalise hard drugs because there will always be drug-takers. If people are being beaten up in the backstreets should we establish clinics where they can be attacked in hygienic conditions? Of course not.

When the child is disabled

Various tests are now available to detect disability in the womb in pregnancy. The principal tests are:

1. Chorionic villus sampling (CVS) – not widely available, this tests a tiny part of the placenta very early in pregnancy.
2. Alfafetoprotein test (AFP) – widely used, this involves testing a blood sample from the mother at about 16 weeks.
3. Amniocentesis test – generally available, this involves removing some of the amniotic fluid from around the child by syringe at about 18 weeks.
4. Ultrasound scanning – generally available, as well as a useful tool in dating the pregnancy, ultrasound can reveal the development of the child by 'bouncing' soundwaves off the bay to produce a living picture on the screen of a monitor.

However and whenever disability is detected, the child needs help with the difficulties and the family needs support. Abortion does not prevent or help disability. It kills the disabled. Acceptance of abortion on these grounds has led to the killing of newborn disabled children who are unwanted or rejected. To kill a child because he or she is disabled strikes many people as particularly cruel and unfair.

Moreover, prenatal screening is not wholly reliable. It is reckoned that 10% of diagnoses by ultrasound machines are inaccurate. Other tests may reveal spina bifida, for instance, but cannot predict the degree of disability in the born child. As well as resulting in healthy children being put to death, amniocentesis (like CVS) can seriously damage children in the womb and has at least 1% chance of causing miscarriage. Special needs children are still human beings. Should we

	Total abortions	Live births (1,000s)	Illegitimacy rate
1968	23,641	842	8.5%
1974	162,941	840	8.8%
1985	171,873	656	19.2%
1994	166,876	665	32.4%
1996	177,275	650	35.8%
2000	185,375	604	39.5%
2001	186,200	595	40%

Abortion statistics

Source: Office of National Statistics, Crown copyright

discriminate against them? We are all disabled to some extent!

Abortion after rape?

Conception can result from rape, but this is rare. There are surveys covering thousands of cases of rape which report no pregnancy. But it sometimes does happen.

Whether or not pregnancy has resulted, the raped woman needs a lot of help to recover from the terrible experience.

In deciding whether abortion can be part of this help, we must remember that abortion itself is a violation of a woman, and that many women are damaged by it. Some women suffer terribly from post-abortion syndrome which means that an abortion following rape may add to the woman's problems rather than help her recover from them.

While some might think that continuing the pregnancy will remind the woman of the rape, experience often tells a different story. Some women in this situation accept the child as something good coming out of something awful, and

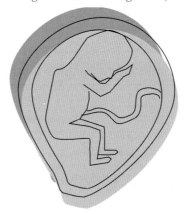

want to keep the child and not, for example, give it away for adoption.

The child, of course, is innocent of any guilt and is just like any other child. It seems unfair to punish the child, condemning him/her to death, because of his/her father's crime. The violence of abortion is no solution to the violence of rape.

Abortion to save the life of the mother?

In years gone by, we are told, the choice between saving the mother or the child was not uncommon. Medical knowledge and science have advanced in recent years to such an extent that this need not be the case in our own days.

There are nowadays a few occasions when the life of the mother is threatened by the pregnancy. This is normally late in pregnancy and, of course, the pregnancy must be ended, otherwise both mother and child will die. But there is no reason to perform an abortion and thereby kill the child. The child can be delivered (by surgery) and given a chance to survive. Children delivered a little over half-way through pregnancy now have a much better chance of survival because of the skill of doctors and the facilities available in Special Baby Care Units.

In this rare situation good medicine can save both mother and baby, and there is now no need to kill either.

■ The above information is from LIFE's web site which can be found at www.lifeuk.org

© LIFE

Widespread ignorance of abortion rights

Women's knowledge about abortion law and practice was shown to be surprisingly poor in a survey published by reproductive health charity Marie Stopes International (MSI).

But when they learnt the true facts, a massive majority (88%) disagreed with the current law and felt that the decision should ultimately rest with the woman.

Presumably, this lack of awareness about abortion is because the subject is rarely discussed openly. Most people only find out the truth when they or somebody close to them needs one. And afterwards, abortion returns to being a taboo subject – an experience best forgotten which we hope we will never need to go through again.

MSI has long contended that 'by perpetuating a conspiracy of silence around abortion, British society does a grave disservice to women.

'Not only does a law that denies a woman's right to make autonomous, informed decisions about her own fertility remain effectively unchallenged in the parliamentary arena, but lack of awareness of treatment options that should be available also has some very real implications for her physical and psychological wellbeing.'

Who decides?

Q. 1 Two doctors have to give written permission for a legal abortion?
(True)
24% said this is correct
33% believed it is just one doctor
33% believed that abortion is legally available solely at the request of the woman.

Q. 2 The consent of a woman's husband or partner is required.
(False)
37% incorrectly thought this was true.

Having established their understanding of legal consent under the 1867 Act, the survey then asked whose consent should be needed. Only 4% agreed with the current legal framework and the massive majority, 88%, believed that the woman should be able to decide for herself. Clearly there would be massive support for law reform if more people knew what the current situation is.

Describing their attitudes to abortion:

- 76% said all women should have the right to an abortion
- 67% said all women should have their abortion funded by the NHS
- 27% said abortion is morally wrong

As these percentages add up to more than 100% and only 11% disagreed that all women should have the right to an abortion, some of those who think abortion is wrong nevertheless support other women's right to choose.

Q. 3 What is the legal time limit? Up to how many weeks of pregnancy can an abortion be legally obtained?
(abortion is available up to 24 weeks in most circumstances but up to term if her life or that of the fetus is seriously threatened)

Up to 12 weeks	32%
UP to 16 weeks	26%
Up to 20 weeks	15%
Up to 24 weeks	13%
Up to 28 weeks	5%
Don't know/refused	9%

It is shocking that so few women, only 13%, knew the correct time limit and that as many as a third believed the time limit was only 12 weeks. Does this mean that some women have not opted for abortion because they wrongly believed they were beyond the legal time limit? (It is also true that nine out of ten abortions are carried out in the first 12 weeks.)

Q. 4 What are the treatment options? Which of these are you aware of?

Emergency contraception* (morning after pill)	92%
Abortion pill	43%
Surgical abortion	75%
Don't know/refused	6%

* Although it is NOT a method of abortion, emergency contraception was included as an option in an attempt to avoid confusion with 'the abortion pill'. Emergency contraceptive pills, also known as

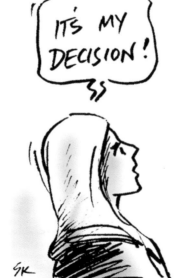

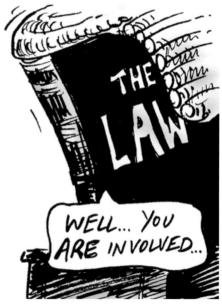

'morning after pills', can prevent a fertilised egg from implanting in the womb if taken within 3 days (72 hours). The pills are available from chemists, doctors and family planning clinics.

The abortion pill, which used to be known as RU486 and now by its brand name Mifepristone, can be used up to nine weeks of pregnancy. It is classified as a legal abortion so has to be carried out under the restrictions of the 1967 Abortion Act. It can only be taken under medically supervised conditions in hospitals or licensed abortion clinics and is not for sale or made available to the public in any other way. This procedure is now referred to as a medical abortion because it only involves the use of drugs, as opposed to a surgical abortion using instruments or equipment to remove the contents of the womb.

Although Mifepristone has been available in this country for more than ten years, the survey showed considerable confusion with 'the morning after pill' when the women who had heard of the abortion pill were asked about the time limit in which it could be used, only 8% correctly said nine weeks. A quarter (24%) said three days, the limit for emergency contraception, and a further 8% said within 24 hours.

Out of those who had heard of surgical abortions, 59% thought that this was possible ONLY under general anaesthetic, showing considerable ignorance of the possible use of local anaesthetic (an injection directly into the cervix to cause numbing and therefore reduction in pain at the mouth of the womb although the patient remains wide awake) and/or the more recently approved use of conscious sedation

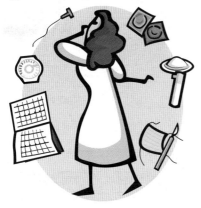

(an intravenous injection of a mix of pain killer and sedative to cause deep relaxation and drowsiness to reduce the discomfort and anxiety).

MSI points out that the vast majority of abortions are still carried out using general anaesthetic in heavily medicalised settings although other procedures have been shown to carry significantly fewer risks for women's health. 'The prevailing culture of silence means that women generally accept what is offered to them, or what they are told they must have – usually a general anaesthetic procedure.'

How common is abortion?

When asked to estimate how many women will have an abortion at some time in their lives, very few women gave the correct answer of one in three. The majority feel that either one in five (30%) or one in 10 (23%) are more likely.

Despite the fact that about five and a half million women have had an abortion in the past 35 years since abortion was made legal in Britain, the lack of awareness of how commonplace the operation is shows how rarely it must be admitted or talked about.

ALRA agrees with the conclusions of MSI that:

The challenge facing British society today is the creation of both a legal framework and a service which reflect women's expectations.

■ A legal framework that recognises and respects that only the woman concerned is competent to make informed decisions about her own fertility regulation

■ A service that is safe, prompt, caring and responsive; offers women choice from the variety of modern treatment options available; and is free at the point of delivery.

What you can do:

■ first of all, check your facts
■ ask friends, relatives and colleagues what they know about abortion law and the treatments available, correct their false perceptions if necessary
■ if you have had a abortion, talk about it with people you know
■ write to your MP about the need for abortion law reform
■ contact your local newspaper or radio station, especially if few abortions are funded by the NHS in your area
■ suggest a talk or discussion on abortion in any association or group you belong to

The independent survey was carried out for MSI by BRMB Social Research. Copies of the report are available from the MSI Marketing Dept, 153-157 Cleveland St, London W1T 6QW. Tel: 020 7574 7356.

■ The above information is from ALRA's *Newsletter*, Issue 82, March 2003. See page 41 for their address details.

© The Abortion Law Reform Association (ALRA)

Abortion FAQs

Information from the ProLife Alliance

Q. Is the ProLife Alliance against all abortion?
A. Yes, we are against the deliberate ending of any innocent human life right from its start when a sperm and an ovum unite to make a new human being. Abortion is also harmful to women, who often regret it and suffer in mind and body.

Q. What about women who have had an abortion?
A. We do not judge or blame or condemn women who have had an abortion. We understand the pressures, the lack of accurate information and support and time to think clearly, which may have led to a rushed and often bitterly regretted decision.

Q. Is the ProLife Alliance against abortion even to save the mother's life?
A. Very rarely an operation to save the mother's life, such as the removal of a cancerous womb, or a damaged fallopian tube in an ectopic pregnancy, must inevitably result in the unwanted side-effect of the baby's death. This is very sad but it is not an abortion, it is not the deliberate ending of a life, it has never been illegal, and no one is against it. In other, still rare, cases, doctors may be able to save mother and baby by letting the pregnancy continue until the baby can survive outside the womb. Improved medical knowledge has practically ended the old choice between saving mother or baby, though there may still be very occasional cases where a difficult choice may need to be made in balancing the mother's health and the baby's.

Q. What if the mother is very young?
A. Apart from the obvious fact that it can never be right to take a child's life, the quick fix of abortion is particularly harmful for very young girls, both mentally and physically.

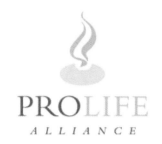

Positive practical help can save the baby's life and the mother's health and happiness.

Q. What if the pregnancy resulted from rape?
A. Abortion does not undo the rape; it adds another horrible experience, leaving the woman feeling doubly a victim. Putting aside the unfairness of an innocent child being killed for her father's crime, there is some evidence that it is better psychologically for the woman if she can be helped to continue the pregnancy, legitimately seeing herself as a heroine who has taken charge of the

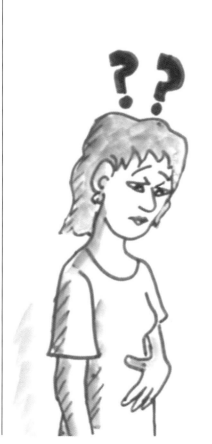

situation and protected her child. She can then if she wishes hand over the baby to loving adoptive parents as a positive closure to her dreadful experience, or choose to keep the baby herself. In real life, as opposed to fiction, violent rape is extraordinarily unlikely to result in pregnancy, and women tend to love their babies even if they hate the father. (One of the worst cruelties of slavery was that children fathered on slaves by their masters were sold separately from their loving mothers.) It is also extremely difficult to prove the truth or falsehood of an allegation of rape. Roe v. Wade, which led to a million abortions a year in the USA, was based on a case where a woman claimed to have been raped but admitted fifteen years later that she had lied. Rape cases make up a very small proportion of the hundreds of thousands of abortions every year in the UK.

Q. What if the baby is disabled?
A. A disabled baby is a human being who needs extra help. Out of about 173,000 abortions in 1999 (the last year for which statistics are available) 1,813 were for suspected handicap. Some of these babies will have been perfectly healthy, others only slightly disabled. What message are we sending to handicapped children and adults and people injured in e.g. road accidents, if we cull pre-born babies as 'sub-standard'? The vast majority given help are as likely to lead happy fulfilled lives as those who think of themselves as able-bodied. Of course if we say that abortion of the handicapped is wrong, we are duty bound to offer help to them and their families.

Q. What about women's rights?
A. We are totally in favour of a woman's rights over her own body, her right to give or refuse consent to sexual intercourse. We are against a woman's 'right' to choose to abort her baby for the same reason as we

are against a man's 'right' to beat his wife, or anyone's 'right' to keep a slave, namely that this infringes the rights of another human being.

Q. If abortion is illegal, won't women die from botched back-street abortions?

A. We are just as much against illegal as against legal abortions, but this question is based on the inaccurate assumption that legalising abortion has saved women's lives. Figures quoted for illegal abortions before 1967 were deliberately exaggerated. The horror stories come from the 1930s and 1940s. After that, and well before the 1967 Abortion Act, deaths recorded as from illegal abortions, from all maternity-related problems (which may of course include illegal abortions not recorded

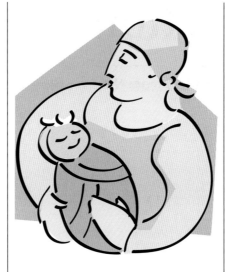

as such) and of women of child-bearing age in general, were all coming down in number at a rate which continued unchanged after the Act. This applies to other

countries in the developed world, regardless of when they made abortion easier (or even in four cases harder) to get. It must be the result of better medicine, probably mainly antibiotics. Most women will not risk an illegal operation, knowing it to be risky, though in fact legal abortions are not as safe as they think. Many women who have legal abortions have complications needing treatment in hospital, many more go to the doctor for physical or psychiatric help, and the increased risk of suicide after abortion compared with giving birth means that more, not fewer, women die.

■ The above information is from ProLife Alliance's web site which can be found at www.prolife.org.uk

© *ProLife Alliance*

LIFE *mourns 35 years of forgotten fathers*

LIFE, the largest pro-life charity in the UK, has called for greater protection of the rights of fathers, in anticipation of the 35th Father's Day since abortion was legalised in the UK.

Since the Abortion Act 1967 was passed, doctors are entitled under section 1(2) to observe the 'actual or foreseeable environment' of the pregnant woman when considering her request for an abortion. However, this provision does not extend to the environment, wishes or feelings of partners.

Patrick Cusworth, LIFE Research and PR Officer, commented that: 'It is ironic that although section 1(1) of the Act allows that the welfare of any existing children may be taken into account when an abortion of a baby under twenty-four weeks is being considered, the rights or opinions of a father can be so easily disregarded by all concerned. Where fathers have gone to court to assert their rights as fathers to be consulted, they have been blocked at every turn. In one notable case, a father was told that he had "no rights whatsoever".

'Cases such as this have meant that there are no circumstances where a man can either protect his own fatherhood or save the life of his unborn child, even if he offers to take over the care of the child after it is born. There is nothing in our legislation that even says that a man has any right even to know of his own fatherhood. However, if the mother decides to give birth, the father is responsible for maintenance until the child reaches the age of 18.

'By marginalising men in pregnancy decisions, abortion trivialises the role of a father in children's lives, and all concerned pay the price: a dead baby, and two parents who are often left devastated by the whole brutal experience. LIFE counsels hundreds of men every year who have fathered babies who were subsequently aborted, and who consequently experience a form of post-abortion trauma. Symptoms of this can be as severe as the loss, grief, depression and guilt suffered by women. Yet our society refuses to allow either parent to weep for the death of their unborn child – even now, with overwhelming evidence of the tragic psychological consequences for both parents, pro-abortion groups still try to deny the existence of post-abortion trauma. Its "pull yourself together" response helps nobody – bar the abortionists who are free to carry out their trade on the next unsuspecting person.

'What these men want is recognition, not subjugation, of their rights and roles as fathers. Many of them feel that such political prejudice is less about a "woman's right to choose" than a man's being forced not to. LIFE calls upon the government to protect men's rights as fathers. The law must adequately reflect the rights of both parents, both before and after birth.'

■ The above information is from LIFE's web site which can be found at www.lifeuk.org

© *LIFE 2003*

Men too

Abortion information for men

Every year, tens of thousands of couples face unplanned pregnancies despite having used a method of family planning. Contraception can fail however careful you are.

About four women in every 10 have an abortion at some time in their lives. Abortion is legal in Britain if two doctors agree that certain criteria are met. Most of these relate to the effect that the pregnancy may have on the mental or physical health of a woman.

BPAS was set up 30 years ago shortly after abortion was legalised to provide a specialist, confidential, non-judgmental service. Today we provide almost 50,000 abortions each year and work closely with the NHS.

What happens at BPAS?

At BPAS, we make every effort for partners to be involved, although they have no legal rights in relation to abortion and our main priority must be the safety and confidentiality of our clients.

Your partner must have two appointments with BPAS, which may involve quite a lot of waiting around for you.

The consultation appointment

■ The first appointment can take

BPAS

British Pregnancy Advisory Service

up to two hours while your partner sees an admin-counsellor and then one of our doctors.

■ You will be able to stay with your partner for most of the time, provided that this is what she wants. At some point during the consultation, however, we will need to see her alone to give her the opportunity for a private discussion.

The abortion appointment

■ We will ask your partner not to eat or drink before treatment if she is having a general anaesthetic. It is important to follow these instructions, otherwise we will have to delay or postpone treatment.

■ Facilities at our clinics (where your partner will have her abortion on the second appointment date) vary a great deal. If you wish to wait for your partner at the clinic, please check parking arrangements as many BPAS premises do not have their own car parks. Drinks and snacks are available at some clinics but not all. Directions to the clinic and a

map will have been given to your partner at the first appointment.

■ Be prepared for more waiting whilst your partner is having her abortion. You will usually be able to stay with her until she is ready for treatment. We will let you know the time we anticipate that she will be able to go home. Usually there is no need for women to stay in the clinic overnight but, if this is necessary, we can provide details of local accommodation for you.

■ We recommend that women have a post-operative check two weeks after their abortion. Usually this can be with a GP, doctor at a family planning clinic or a BPAS consultation centre.

The abortion procedure

Abortion procedures vary according to the stage of the pregnancy. Depending on medical advice, women are able to choose the procedure that they feel is most suitable for them and their circumstances. The procedures are described more fully in the leaflets *Abortion options in early pregnancy*, *Abortion options after 14 weeks of pregnancy*.

These are available at BPAS consultation centres, or from BPAS head office on 01564 793 225.

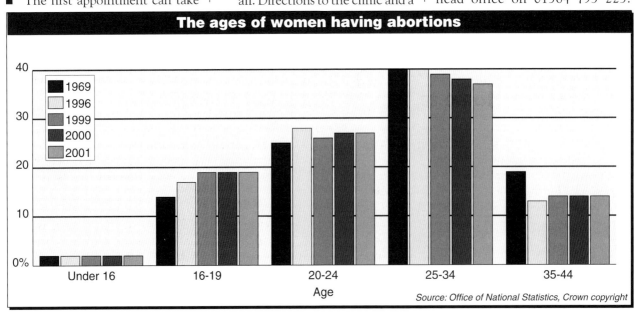

The ages of women having abortions

Legend: 1969, 1996, 1999, 2000, 2001

Age: Under 16, 16-19, 20-24, 25-34, 35-44

Source: Office of National Statistics, Crown copyright

Further information is also available on the BPAS website www.bpas.org

Abortion procedures, especially in the early weeks of pregnancy, are very safe but obviously no clinical procedure is entirely without risk. Your partner should discuss her choices of treatment, and any possible complications and side effects, with a doctor or nurse practitioner, before she makes her decision.

Short-term effects

One of the highest risks after an abortion is infection. All our clients are given a course of antibiotics to minimise this risk. Women are also advised to avoid sexual intercourse for two weeks after treatment, and to use sanitary towels instead of tampons.

It is usual for women to experience some bleeding for several days after an abortion. Exactly what your partner can expect will be explained before she leaves the clinic as it depends on her procedure. However, if she has any concerns over bleeding she can call the BPAS Post Treatment Support Line on 00800 6655 5566.*

* Please note: Some mobile telephones block 00800 numbers, so you may not be able to get through to this number using your mobile phone. If you experience difficulties, please use an ordinary telephone.

Similarly, if she feels unwell she should seek medical advice. It is always better to seek advice than worry unnecessarily.

After treatment, some women find that their hormone levels swing quite dramatically whilst their bodies adjust. This may result in mood changes and it is common for women to feel a bit sensitive and irritable. This is perfectly normal, but you may find that your partner needs extra support and reassurance.

There is a slight risk of continuing pregnancy following the abortion. If your partner is still experiencing the symptoms of pregnancy two to three weeks after her abortion she should seek advice from her doctor.

Longer-term effects

There is very little risk to future fertility unless a woman contracts an infection and it is not properly treated. This is why it is so important for your partner to follow our aftercare advice.

There is no evidence that abortion causes long-term depression or trauma. After an abortion, some women feel a sense of loss, even if they believe their decision was right. Others may feel relief. Feelings after an abortion depend on individual circumstances. Try to take the lead from your partner and help her in the way that she feels is most supportive.

■ The above information is from British Pregnancy Advisory Service's web site which can be found at www.bpas.org

© British Pregnancy Advisory Service (BPAS)

Questions men ask us

Can I tell my friends?

It may be useful for you and your partner to discuss where you would like to find some additional support. She may find it helpful to share her feelings with female friends, and equally you may want to talk to a male friend. Try to agree together who you will talk to, including friends and family so you both know who is aware of your situation.

Will she feel differently about sex?

There is no reason why an abortion will necessarily affect a woman's feelings about sex, but when contraception has failed this in itself might make her feel insecure. Sometimes women fear that nothing is 'safe' and they might become pregnant again.

How soon can we have sex?

Vaginal penetration should be avoided for two weeks after the abortion. If you both find it impossible to wait, use a condom to help prevent infection.

She had the abortion two weeks ago but is still upset. When are things going to be back to how they should be?

After an abortion, women can experience a variety of emotions and feelings, some of which may appear contradictory. They may feel relieved but also quite sad. Sometimes there are feelings of loss but these normally decrease with time. All women are different and there is no standard amount of time that it takes for a woman to put her abortion experience behind her. BPAS can provide post-abortion counselling at any time after an abortion.

I can't seem to say the right thing

It can be hard for a man to discuss an unplanned pregnancy. It may feel as though you are pushing a particular view if you keep raising the matter. Equally if you avoid the issue it may seem that you are distant or uncaring. The only guide here is to be led by your partner, and ask her what she wants. However, be prepared that what she wants may well vary from day to day – even from hour to hour.

I feel helpless and excluded from what's going on

It is not surprising that some men feel isolated when their partner has an abortion. To some extent this is unavoidable given that the final decisions about the future of a pregnancy must ultimately rest with the pregnant woman. You can ask your partner how she would like you to support her and, by respecting her wishes, you will be doing the best you can.

This is affecting our relationship. What can we do?

It can be very difficult to cope with an unplanned pregnancy, particularly if you both have different expectations from your relationship. One of the hardest situations can be when there is a difference of opinion over continuing the pregnancy. It may be helpful to seek professional help if you find that your relationship is suffering. Relate can provide professional counselling and can be contacted on 01788 573241 or www.relate.org.uk

Teenage pregnancies

Why we are failing

As SPUC intensifies its campaign against the abortion-inducing morning-after pill, challenging the policy of targeting teenage girls, including those under the age of 16, remains a central concern. Many people find it hard to understand why giving teenage girls more and more access to contraceptives, surgical abortions and the morning-after pill, has not led to a reduction in teenage pregnancies. Dr David Paton of Nottingham University looks at how current policies are failing.

Teenage pregnancy and abortion rates in the UK are amongst the highest in the developed world and the Government has vowed to reduce conception rates amongst under-18s by 50% by 2010. Showing a singular lack of imagination, the Government's Teenage Pregnancy Strategy is concentrating on increasing young people's access to confidential (i.e. without parental knowledge) family planning services. Amongst the most controversial measures are that all young pregnant women should have early access to NHS-funded abortion and that youngsters under the age of 16 should have access to the morning-after pill at supermarkets and at schools.

For many people, family planning is an obvious solution. If more youngsters who are having sex used contraception, then surely we would have fewer pregnancies. In fact, you may be surprised to learn that the majority of youngsters who get pregnant were using some form of contraception already; they became pregnant because the contraception failed.[1]

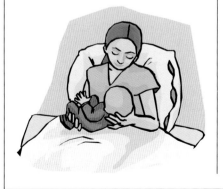

In order to understand the factors that really contribute to teenage pregnancy, we need to ask: why is it that some youngsters decide to have sex and others don't? For some it may be peer pressure, for others the influence of drink or perhaps just curiosity. One of the biggest factors in the decision is the youngster's attitude to pregnancy. Some teenagers actively want to get pregnant, and providing family planning is unlikely to change anything for this group. Other youngsters are keen to avoid pregnancy. Providing family planning makes these youngsters believe they are less likely to get pregnant and, as a result, more of them are likely to have sex. We are sometimes told, 'Young people are going to have sex anyway – nothing will change that'. Well, think about the following scenario. Say 100 youngsters have decided to have sex. Now say we were to remove all access to any form of family planning. Would all 100 still decide to have sex? Of course not! Those who want to get pregnant will still have sex. Some of the others will too, perhaps due to ignorance or peer pressure. However, at least some of those who are really keen to avoid pregnancy will now decide to abstain from sex.

The bottom line is that providing family planning in schools is likely to have two effects. Those girls who would have had sex anyway are less likely to get pregnant because they have greater access to contraceptives. However, the number of pregnancies among those girls who start to have sex as a result of providing family planing is likely to increase, because if they weren't having sex at all they wouldn't get pregnant. We can only judge the overall effect by looking at the evidence. In fact, my research, recently published in the *Journal of Health Economics*, shows that increasing access to family planning for youngsters simply has not reduced teenage pregnancy rates.[2] Many other papers have some to a similar conclusion. In the case of the morning-after pill, a study published in the *British Medical Journal* found that youngsters who were prescribed the morning-after pill were more likely to go on to have abortions at a later stage.[3] Rather worryingly, little or no research has examined the impact of these types of policies on rates of sexually transmitted diseases.

There are two possible ways to interpret the finding that family planning has not reduced teenage pregnancies. One is that access to family planning removes a restraint on those teenagers who would otherwise not engage in sex. The other interpretation is that access to family planning has no effect on youngsters' behaviour at all. Either way, it seems very likely that recent proposals to provide condoms and the morning-after pill to youngsters at school without their parents knowing will help in reducing teenage pregnancies.

If you think you've heard this somewhere before, then you probably have. In 1992, the last Conservative Government announced its intention to increase access to family planning with the aim of reducing teenage pregnancies amongst under-16s by 50% by the year 2000. What was the result? Well, attendance by under-16s at family planning clinics rose by 143.6% between 1992 and 2000. Prescriptions of the morning-after pill to this age group at family planning clinics rose by 284.8%. Over the same period, the conception rate amongst under-16s went down from 8.4 per 1000 girls in 1992 to 8.3 per 1000 in 2000!

The myth that providing family planning and the morning-after pill for under-16s without parental knowledge is an easy way to reduce teenage pregnancy should be challenged at every opportunity. Our children deserve something better than an out-of-date approach that simply doesn't work.

Our children deserve something better than an out-of-date approach that simply doesn't work

References
1   Churchill, D. et al (2000), 'Consultation Patterns and Provision of Contraception in General Practice Before Teenage Pregnancy: case-control study', *British Medical Journal*, 2, 1, 486-9.
2   Paton, David (2002). 'The Economics of Family Planning and Underage Conceptions', *Journal of Health Economics*, 21, 2 (March), 27-45.
3   Churchill et al. op. cit.

■ The above information is from the *Pro-Life Times*, produced by SPUC. See page 41 for their address details.
© *SPUC*

One in three

Abortion, often the subject of secretiveness and widely thought of as relatively rare, is actually a commonplace experience for women in Britain. The day-to-day reality seems at odds with the present state of the law on abortion. Here six women tell their stories

It is a commonly quoted statistic – that one in four women will have an abortion during their lifetime. In fact, according to the Royal College of Obstetricians and Gynaecologists, that is an underestimate. At least a third of British women will have an abortion by the age of 45 (excluding Northern Ireland, where abortion is still illegal). In 2001, there were 186,000 legal abortions carried out in England and Wales (17 per 1,000 women aged 15-44). That figure remains fairly constant from year to year, although there was a peak in 1996, coinciding with a health scare over the pill.

Under the terms of the Abortion Act of 1967, termination is legal up to the 24th week of pregnancy, subject to approval from two doctors. To 'qualify' for an abortion, a woman must prove that having a baby would cause her or her family greater physical or mental damage than not having one. Effectively, this places the power to decide in the hands of the medical profession, and does not provide women with the legal right to choose. The UK differs from other European nations and the US in this respect. 'The current law tells you that there are very few politicians who will pay anything more than lip service to the idea of women's rights,' says Dr Ellie Lee, editor of *Abortion: Whose Right?*

While in practice many doctors interpret the law liberally, they are nonetheless able to block access to services on the basis of moral opposition. A survey conducted by Marie Stopes International (MSI) in 1999 found that 18% of GPs were opposed to abortion, yet they do not have to declare this objection to patients. According to Alice Richardson, chairwoman of the National Abortion Campaign, women report numerous incidents of 'notes lost, decisions delayed and confidentiality broken' by doctors. Many women prefer to refer to a specialist abortion provider, such as the British Pregnancy Advisory Service (BPAS) or MSI – both of which are charities. If seeking an NHS abortion, however, a woman initially has to go through her surgery or family planning clinic.

She may then face a second hurdle: NHS provision for abortions is patchy, resulting in what Richardson describes as 'abortion by postcode'. The amount of funding made available for abortion varies widely from borough to borough: in 2001, for example, 96% of abortions in North Cumbria were NHS-funded;

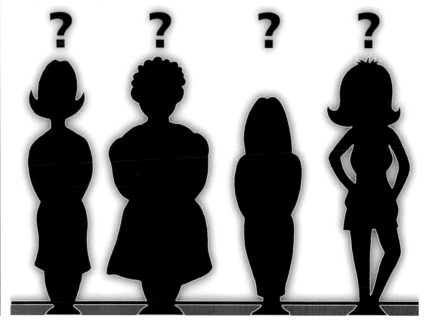

in Dorset, the figure was 61%; in Kingston and Richmond, in Surrey, meanwhile, only 50%. Health authorities set different time ceilings on abortions – in some areas, they are refused to women who are more than 11 weeks pregnant. Waiting lists – even for an initial appointment – are commonplace. Much of the burden of abortion provision is undertaken by charities such as MSI and BPAS. In 2001, 33% of NHS abortions were contracted to such organisations, while 24% of all abortions were private – at a cost, on average, of £400.

Public opinion polls show high rates of approval for abortion, but there is still a minority that disagrees. The Society for the Protection of the Unborn Child campaigns on this issue and seeks a tightening of the current law. Its education officer, Katherine Hampton, says, 'It is too easy for people to get abortions and I don't think they are given enough information – at the time they are considering abortion and earlier, at school.'

Pro-choice campaigners, meanwhile, advocate greater honesty in this area: 'Accidental pregnancy is so predictable, and so much a part of having a sexual relationship,' says Lee. 'We are dishonest in saying we can be 100% in control. It is simply not true.' A spokesperson for MSI describes the current abortion law as 'paternalistic, way out of date, and long due for reform'.

Mary Williamson, 66, Colchester
It was in the 1980s, I was 44 or 45. The cap failed and I found, to my absolute horror, that I was pregnant. I'd come off the pill because of a health scare and thought that there was less and less chance that I would become pregnant. It was pretty awful – the whole idea of having another child was totally unplanned and unlooked for. I had one child who was then 19 and didn't want any more. I'm married and we discussed it. I told my mother and there was no disapproval at all – if I'd have had to go privately, she would have helped me. My daughter was in America at the time – I can't remember when I told her, but it certainly wasn't a secret. I had a national health

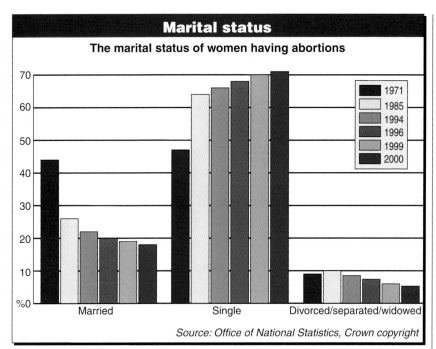

Marital status
The marital status of women having abortions

Legend: 1971, 1985, 1994, 1996, 1999, 2000

Source: Office of National Statistics, Crown copyright

abortion, which was very quick – but it was traumatic because of the decision to make, and also because I'm old enough to remember when it would have been a fate worse then death to need an abortion.

I was pleasantly surprised at the availability. I think I was six weeks pregnant when I realised, and a couple of weeks later I'd had the abortion. My GP wasn't too hot, but he did put me on to a consultant, who was brilliant – no judgmental remarks or anything. I must have been quite worried at the time, but looking back it was a relatively straightforward procedure, which was almost totally due to having a very caring consultant. I overheard him saying to a nurse, 'This is what the 1967 Abortion Act was all about.'

Public opinion polls show high rates of approval for abortion, but there is still a minority that disagrees

---

The doctor who referred me to the consultant was fairly old and I had to bring it up – he probably wanted me to say the word 'abortion' rather than him. In hospital, they kept asking whether I wanted to go

ahead, but I guess they had to in case I changed my mind. I had it on a Wednesday and went back to work the next Monday. A year later, I had a sterilisation, just to make sure it didn't happen again.

I've absolutely no regrets, I'll always remember the enormous feeling of relief when I woke up in hospital. I've never been mentally ill, or any of the things they say you are going to be – I'm not walking around damaged beyond repair. I'm very upfront and open about it, and I feel it should be talked about. It is a private and shameful thing in many people's eyes – not, I hasten to add, in mine. People are a little bit shocked and surprised when I talk about it; they take it for granted that I'm against abortion, partly because of my age and partly because I appear very 'respectable' – we live in a small village and I was a lecturer in further education. The perception is that people like me aren't supposed to have abortions.

Sally Helliwell, 35, London
I was 23 and about to go to university. Though I was in a relationship and living with the bloke, I definitely didn't want to have children. I was on the pill, so it was a bit of a shock. But I didn't really consider any other option – there was no question, either for me or for my partner at the time. I never had any dilemmas about it – it was just a practical thing to do. I think it makes a big difference if you

are in a situation where you might want children, but you aren't quite sure. That might have an impact on your decision.

I approached the whole thing in a very matter-of-fact way. We made an appointment at the doctor's and had to go through the rigmarole of getting two doctors' consent, although fortunately it was fairly straightforward and I didn't get any hassle. It was very early on when I found out – seven weeks – and I had to wait to have the abortion, they said it was too small to do it any earlier.

There are two images I remember of going to hospital. Seeing this girl I knew in the waiting room and lying on the operating table waiting for the general anaesthetic to take effect. I can't really remember any of the details – but why would you? I don't remember getting my teeth taken out, either. Even giving birth, which I did 18 months ago, is fading from my memory pretty quickly.

It is very different finding out you've made a mistake and working out how you're going to deal with it, then wanting a child, getting pregnant and looking forward to having one

---

I did have an instance when I was 19 and thought that I was pregnant, and went to see a doctor who made it very clear, even before I had the tests, that she was anti-abortion. I was scared stiff that I was pregnant and was insinuating that I wasn't going to have the baby. She made it clear that it wasn't an option as far as she was concerned.

So when I was pregnant at 23, I thought that was going to happen again, but it didn't. My impression from that is that it very much depends on the doctor – you can be lucky or unlucky. When it comes to practicalities, most people think abortion is OK, but that can change when you

talk about it in the abstract as a moral issue; then there's this whole thing that women are supposed to be traumatised by it. And the whole process of doctors ticking boxes to say that you'll be more traumatised by having a child than if you don't, to say that your mental health is at risk if you go through with the pregnancy – that puts across the idea that somehow you are doing something you shouldn't be doing. Or something that will affect you in the future, when really there is no reason why it should.

I was very confident about what I wanted to do. It was a long time ago and I haven't really thought about it since. I didn't even think about it when I had my child. It is very different finding out you've made a mistake and working out how you're going to deal with it, then wanting a child, getting pregnant and looking forward to having one.

Sue Hulbert, 40, Leeds

It was May 12 2000 when I had the abortion, a date that is fixed in my mind. The next day that sticks is November 19, because that's when my child was due. Whatever anybody says, there will always be a life missing from my life. I hope and pray that one day I will see him and that he will forgive me.

I was involved in a relationship that had problems, but the baby was planned. Every relationship goes through rocky patches – I just didn't know how rocky. As soon as I got pregnant, my partner refused to talk about the baby. Things between us got worse, strained, we started to argue a lot and he became quite aggressive. In the end, we had an enormous argument and I remember screaming at him, 'I don't want you or your baby.' On the day we should have gone to the hospital for the first pregnancy consultation, we actually went and spoke about abortion.

The hospital made it very easy for me. Although the first consultant did say he wouldn't do it, he put me in touch with

someone who would. Within a fortnight, I was booked in. My pre-abortion meeting gave me no indication that the abortion was going to cause me any damage, either mentally or physically. On the morning I went in, I was distraught. Even up to that point, I had an idea that I would never go through with it. But I went in, was examined, given a pessary, and two hours later I had the abortion.

I woke up in tears – I knew that I'd done the wrong thing. I had a haemorrhage – which was frightening and painful – and another one four weeks later. But, mentally, the problems became more debilitating. The overarching thought in my mind was that I had killed my child. I felt so guilty, I lost all confidence, all my self-esteem, and I wasn't able to do my job. In the end, last December I took an overdose, because I'd decided my life wasn't worth anything. I didn't feel worthy of being a mother to my two kids [from an earlier relationship]: I thought if they ever found out about the baby, they would hate me, and because I was so depressed and crying all the time, I wasn't being a proper mother to them. I spent a long time after that in a hospital psychiatric unit. In the meantime I've had counselling from the British Victims of Abortion [a helpline for those experiencing physical and emotional difficulties after an abortion].

The thing that makes me angry is that I was never told what the side-effects might be, by anybody. I was so weak and I was put under pressure by my partner, who had lowered my self-confidence, anyway. I felt as though I couldn't cope with any-

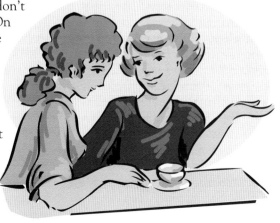

thing. You are in a very vulnerable state, it's a time when you need guidance and structure – and it simply wasn't there.

Without a doubt, I would have been better off having that baby. However many problems I could have had being pregnant, I didn't know I would have far more not having that child. I've had nightmares – I've seen foetuses in hospital kidney bowls, crowds of people shouting at me that I'm a murderer, puréed foetuses being splattered on windows. I have difficulty with other people's two-year-olds – it makes social interaction very hard. I lost work, money – you can't describe the cost of it, or the frustration when people don't understand what you are trying to tell them.

Anonymous, 32, London

I was 27 and had been going out with someone for three months. I found out I was pregnant after we broke up. It was a split condom. I never told my ex, I had no desire to – he's the sort of person who, instead of making me feel better, would have needed me to reassure him. I felt awful finding out I was pregnant. I didn't want to be, it was really horrible. I went to my GP and was really scared: you hear so many horror stories about doctors refusing abortions, and I knew that, if he did refuse, I wouldn't be able to afford one privately. But he was actually really good and referred me to a hospital within a week. Then I had to wait four weeks to have my operation, which was just awful. Not for one moment did I think I was doing the wrong thing, but waiting put me in a state of temporary paralysis. I just wanted it to be over – I couldn't move on, get on with anything. It was a horrible time, going through this so soon after the break-up of a relationship. I couldn't sleep, I couldn't eat – it wasn't good.

I felt stupid being in that position. I'm an intelligent person and I felt like I should have known better. You still think, 'God, I'm so stupid, how could I have got into this position?' Even though I wouldn't think that of anyone else, I thought it about me.

A friend came to the hospital with me and the actual termination was fine. You turn up in the morning and are home by lunchtime, watching videos in the afternoon. When I woke up from the operation, I instantly knew I wasn't pregnant any more – I felt a bit weird, but mostly I just felt relief. I've never felt at all guilty about it, and now I just don't think about it. The only thing I regret is that I was ever in that position in the first place.

I would never tell my mum, it would upset her and she doesn't need to know. I don't regret what I did, but it is still not really acceptable to talk about. You wouldn't think that one in three women has an abortion. There is a lot of stigma attached, and the anti-abortionists like to claim the moral high ground. Plus we're not very good at talking about sex generally – and abortion is one of those things that is supposed to happen to other people.

I felt stupid being in that position. I'm an intelligent person and I felt like I should have known better. You still think, 'God, I'm so stupid, how could I have got into this position?'

Anonymous 24-year-old

It was three years ago. I was at university. At the time, I was very stressed because I was having problems with my family and it was interfering with my studies. My doctor put me on antidepressants and told me they would stop me getting pregnant as well. A month after that, I got pregnant. As soon as I found out, I knew I wanted a termination. At no point did I feel I wanted a child – it just wasn't right for me at the time. I was in what turned out to be a long-term relationship, but at that point we hadn't known each other long.

I was referred to a private clinic on the NHS and had the termination. I was lucky; I know that's not the case for everybody – in my area there

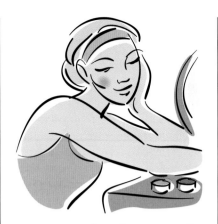

is not very good NHS provision. But part of that was that my doctor realised she'd made a very big mistake, so from then on it went very smoothly.

I didn't tell my family, but my mother is quite nosy and she went through my bag and found a letter. My family went completely mad. It was only then, facing other people's extreme opinions, that I was affected badly. It wasn't the abortion itself, but the reactions of my family that made it difficult – being told by them that I had killed, that I was a murderer. It really upset me. I was studying, away from home, a poor student, and my family messed it up for a few months, made it difficult to concentrate because of endless phone calls and arguments. They said it was because they're strict Muslims, but I know now that views within the religion vary quite a lot, especially on early abortions. It may have been a cultural issue as well for my family – it just wasn't considered acceptable to have an abortion.

But I was quite confident about it at the time, and I still am. I felt that I had a right to do what I did. Purely on an emotional level, it was clear to me from the beginning that this wasn't for me, that I didn't want to be controlled by children I didn't want, that this wasn't a future I wanted at that stage. I thought I had done the adult thing, and it seemed that what my family wanted was for me to be like a child, allow my life to be shaped by circumstances rather than me having agency in my life. It doesn't bother me what they think. What bothers me is that they got in my way and made things much harder for me. I respect anyone who wouldn't choose abortion for themselves. What I don't respect is someone ruining another person's life by telling them that they can't have one.

Anne Quesney, 36, London
About four years ago, I had a total accident, a failure of contraception when a condom split, and suddenly found myself pregnant. I decided to have an abortion because I don't want to have children, full stop. It's something my partner and I decided long ago, so for me it was the only solution. I never thought that decision was right or wrong. It's just a choice women make, and that was it. There were no kind of moral considerations, it was just a practical solution.

I went to the doctor and told him that I thought I was pregnant and wanted an abortion. He was very supportive, so everything happened straightforwardly and very quickly –

I was so adamant about my decision that it made things easier. I was sent to a Marie Stopes clinic, but it was paid for on the NHS. I think I was extremely lucky – I was living in a borough that is known to have one of the worst track records in terms of NHS abortions.

I only had a local anaesthetic – by choice, I didn't feel the need to be totally put out – so I remember the termination clearly. It is a very quick process, a very simple operation, so I don't think there is a need for people to have a general anaesthetic. I think they do it because most women don't want to be conscious. It was over in minutes. You feel slight discomfort – it's not exactly a picnic – but in a sense it's not that much worse than a visit to the dentist. I had a few cramps afterwards, but I assume that was normal. My partner picked me up, and two hours later I was home.

The feeling was relief, straight away. I didn't want to have a child – it was the only solution. There are a lot of women who don't want children; for those who do, it seems a really strange concept, but for those who don't it is totally acceptable. My life carried on. There was no traumatic experience or psychological hang-ups or whatever.

Before I had an abortion, I wasn't aware of the legal situation in this country. It did shock me [that two doctors had to agree to the termination], as I didn't feel I was able to exercise my right over my own body. I can't say I was treated badly in any way, but it's a time when quite a lot of woman can feel vulnerable. I've never come across anyone who told me it was the wrong thing to do – and, in any case, I know it was the right thing, so it doesn't really matter.

© Guardian Newspapers Limited 2003

Manifestations of post-abortion trauma

Some or many of these symptoms may be displayed by the woman who has had an abortion and is experiencing trauma. Keep in mind, many women do not break denial and begin the healing process until seven to ten years after the abortion. These manifestations may occur much sooner and she may seek help for one of these problems without revealing her abortion.

- Low self-esteem
- Depression
- Guilt
- Grief
- Suicidal ideation (in the USA 1,800 to 4,000 calling Suicide Anonymous in a 35-month period had prior abortions. Research by Meta Uchtman, Suicide Anonymous in Ohio.)
- Broken relationships
- Anger
- Flashbacks
- Drug/alcohol abuse
- Sexual dysfunction or promiscuity
- Eating disorder (Anorexia, Bulimia)
- Phobias
- Atonement or replacement baby (many women become pregnant within 1 year of the abortion. Emergency Pregnancy Counsellors report that as many as 50% of their clients have had a previous abortion.)
- Fear for her surviving children

- Inability to express emotions
- Psychic numbing
- Possible physical pain (Psychogenic/Psychosomatic pain such as cramping and cervical pain.)
- Difficult labours
- Premature deliveries
- Repeated miscarriages
- Infertility
- Sleep disturbances (baby dreams, auditory hallucinations of an infant crying, nightmares.)
- Hyper alertness
- Trouble concentrating
- Avoidance of activities that remind her of children/abortion/pregnancy
- Lost relationships
- Self-punishment
- Anxiety in subsequent pregnancies
- Creation of phantom child
- Fascination with children and birth which could become an obsession. (She may fixate on a child of a similar age to hers or fixate on a doll or some object that weighs what her aborted child would have weighed.)

■ The above information is from the organisation British Victims of Abortion (BVA). See page 41 for their address details.

© British Victims of Abortion (BVA)

Tough life choices

By Eleanor Lee

The news that a woman is planning to sue the NHS for the mental distress she experienced following her abortion should not surprise us – this is not the first time action against an abortion provider has been threatened. In 1999 a woman who had had an abortion issued high court proceedings against a clinic and two of its doctors. In 2001, a mother of six threatened to sue an abortion provider for failing to give her adequate counselling. What happened?

When such women tell their stories it is heart-rending. But does it follow that doctors should warn women in advance that they may feel terrible after an abortion? And should they be made to pay when women say they were not warned enough?

> ## When women request an abortion we are making a choice – and should therefore take responsibility for its outcome

Anti-abortion organisations answer yes to both these questions. In both the US and Britain, they have made the issue of mental distress following abortion central to their activities and arguments. They call it 'post-abortion syndrome'.

One counsellor from Life said: 'Post-abortion syndrome is what happens to a woman when she's had an abortion, she hasn't recognised she is traumatised by it, she's pushed it under and hasn't been allowed to grieve, and she gets post-abortion stress.' On this basis, Life offers women post-abortion counselling and argues that women should sue abortion providers on the grounds that they were not warned about such feelings in advance.

The woman currently in the news is being supported by Life. Her case is not driven by grief alone. It is part of Life's political strategy. In 1998 Jack Scarisbrick, the Life national chairman, said: 'We want women who have suffered either physical or mental trauma as a result of abortion to contact us. We will encourage them to take the doctors responsible to court.'

At the moment women who request abortion are informed that, for the vast majority, there is no risk that their mental health will be damaged. This is not because doctors are reckless, but because they are following guidelines from the Royal College of Obstetricians and Gynaecologists. The college is not reckless either; its guidelines draw on a review of all the published research evidence, and conclude that 'only a small minority of women experience any long-term, adverse psychological sequelae after abortion'.

The aftermath of abortion is a well-established field of research. The research has not been dominated by the pro-choice lobby, whatever Life might claim. As part of his campaign against abortion, President Reagan commissioned a review by the then surgeon general Everett Koop about its effects on health. His reasoning was that opposition to abortion would be boosted by the finding that abortion was bad for women's health. In the event, even though Koop was well known for his strongly anti-abortion views, the inquiry found that its mental health risks were 'minuscule from a public health perspective'.

There are always exceptions. Most women do not experience very negative feelings, but some do. The problem is, how can an abortion provider be expected to predict this? If doctors and others played safe when counselling women, and emphasised the experience of the minority, what would this mean for the majority of women who find abortion to be a difficult choice, but the right one? Should they sue for being 'over counselled'?

Providers of a medical service can only base the information they give on the best available evidence. When women request an abortion we are making a choice – and should therefore take responsibility for its outcome. If in the end it turns out to be the wrong choice we might seek counselling to feel better. But the issue should go no further – we cannot blame anyone but ourselves.

> ## Most women do not experience very negative feelings, but some do. The problem is, how can an abortion provider be expected to predict this?

While the law in Britain does not provide for 'abortion on request', most abortions currently take place on the assumption that reproductive decisions are private ones, best made by those who will bear the consequences. The idea that someone else is liable when we feel bad after the exercise of choice is tantamount to saying we are not capable of making the choice – which is precisely why the notion of 'post-abortion syndrome' is so attractive to opponents of legal abortion.

The claim that more should be done to respond to the possibility of negative psychological responses is not really about best practice in abortion care. It is about degrading the notion that women are responsible adults who can act autonomously when making decisions about their reproductive lives.

Dr Eleanor Lee is a sociologist at Southampton University and is author of a forthcoming book, *Inventing Post Abortion Trauma*.
© *Guardian Newspapers Limited 2003*

Why abortion is bad for your mental health

The procedure, says the doctor, is perfectly harmless. The patient complies. Later, however, she returns and says that it has, in fact, made her ill. Nonsense, says the doctor: you must have been ill in the first place. I wasn't, she says. Well, you're ill now, says the doctor; and, since my operation can't possibly make anyone ill, you must have been ill beforehand.

Gillian Penny of the Royal College of Obstetricians and Gynaecologists recently made the gloriously sweeping statement that women who had abortions did not usually suffer psychological problems unless they were already disturbed.

Her remarks came in response to the news that a young woman was planning to sue the NHS for post-abortion psychological trauma. Dr Penny was not the doctor who performed the operation, but she felt able to say: 'I would suggest that this woman perhaps did have pre-existing psychological problems.'

It is a tenet of post-feminist liberalism that abortion is good for you – your foremothers fought for it, that's why. So any evidence that it might have a negative effect on some women is inadmissible.

By Anne Atkins

But common sense tells us that some post-abortion psychological trauma is so likely as to be almost inevitable, for numerous reasons. Suspend, for a moment, your ideology. For most of history, to induce abortion has been a crime inspiring the deepest moral outrage; whatever we think now of these earlier values, is it likely that, in one generation, we could eradicate all guilt at something so recently regarded with such revulsion?

> **Common sense tells us that some post-abortion psychological trauma is so likely as to be almost inevitable, for numerous reasons**

Moreover, every reader probably knows at least one woman who was initially horrified to discover herself pregnant, only to give birth to a child on whom she subsequently doted. If despair followed by delight is such a common feature of childbearing, isn't it at least a possibility that some women, having terminated their pregnancies, will later have regrets?

In fact, there is evidence aplenty. In 1989, the journal *Psychotherapy and Psychosomatics* followed 83 post-abortion patients, and found 30 suffering 'anniversary reactions', often psychosomatic symptoms, on the date either of the abortion or when the baby should have been born. In 1992, Zolese and Blacker (*British Journal of Psychiatry*) summarised previous research to discover a 'marked, severe or persistent psychiatric illness' in an average of 10 per cent of post-abortive women.

In 1996, Kitamura (*Psychotherapy and Psychosomatics*) demonstrated the link between abortion and ante-natal depression in subsequent pregnancies. In the same year, Gissler et al. (*British Medical Journal*) reported that a woman's risk of suicide trebles after an abortion (whereas it halves after childbirth).

Can all this be swept away, on the grounds that these women were

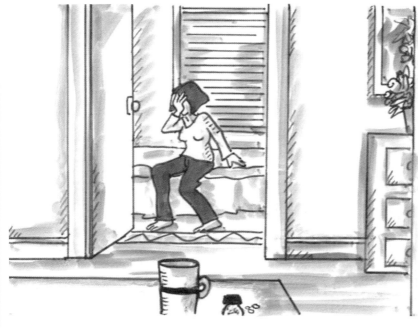

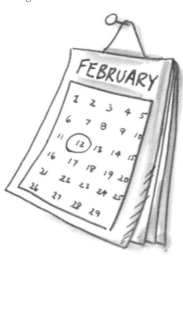

already unstable? Are women who have abortions statistically more likely to be psychologically vulnerable, for instance? Here, the findings are even more disturbing. In 2001, Cagnacci and Volpe (*Human Reproduction*) discovered a seasonal pattern in abortions mirroring seasonal suicide (peaking in May and dipping in November), suggesting that women are more likely to seek abortion when their mood is temporarily low. This helps explain why some women may regret an abortion, after their seasonally depressed mood has passed.

More worrying still, as far back as 1972 (*Psychotherapy and Psychosomatics*), research showed that a previous history of psychiatric illness meant that a woman was more likely to be counselled to abort. But if it is known that abortion can exacerbate depression, surely vulnerable women should be warned of the possible psychological dangers of the operation? Abortion is supposed to be about choice. Genuine choice is informed.

The complaint currently being made against the NHS is that the patient in question was not told. As it happens, she works in the health service and knows it is good practice to give information of the risks of

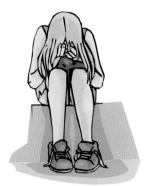

any operation. The need for such information is surely more compelling if the operation is not medically necessary. What possible motive can there be for silence on the subject?

Three reasons suggest themselves. The tackiest and most obvious is financial. Half the abortions in this country are done through private clinics. Doctors may find the operation distasteful, but there is no denying that it is lucrative.

The second is the wording of the 1967 Abortion Act. Abortion is still illegal unless two doctors agree that the risk to the mother's mental or physical health is greater if the pregnancy is continued. As we all know, almost any two busy doctors will sign the wretched thing: if she doesn't want to have the baby, it is presumably better for her mental health not to. On the other hand, if

the evidence shows that abortion can endanger her mental health more than having an unwanted baby, this blows an enormous hole in the Act – or rather the way it is interpreted – and makes all the doctors look like asses, or worse.

Lastly, of course, there is political correctness. You can't question abortion, even though some of the risks are well established. One study, using data from the Office of National Statistics, has estimated that there are already 16,000 women in England and Wales who have developed breast cancer as a direct result of abortion, and this could rise to a total of 300,000 by 2023. Abortion, however, is beyond debate: a woman's right to choose. But is it a free choice?

How many young women are driven, metaphorically as well as literally, to the clinic by someone else? Probably the most frightening discovery of all (*Psychotherapy and Psychosomatics*, 1989) is that women instigate only 30 per cent of abortions. The rest are suggested by parents (seven per cent), friends (10 per cent), doctors (20 per cent) and (an appalling 33 per cent) partners – partners who will not suffer the adverse effects.

Coping with termination

Information from the National Youth Agency

Some facts about abortion

- 1 in 5 pregnancies in the UK end in termination
- 90% of all abortions take place in the first 12 weeks of pregnancies
- Over half of all pregnancies in under-16s end in abortion

Abortion is a sensitive issue and is in fact illegal in some cultures and countries. It is legal in the UK but on the grounds of religious belief, it is illegal in the Republic of Ireland. Anti-abortion campaigners ask the question of whether or not the foetus is alive, does it have an individual right to life and does the woman have the right to choose whether or not she continues with a pregnancy.

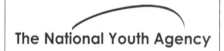

Abortion and religion

It is often people with a committed religious viewpoint who oppose abortion, although some religions are more tolerant than others when it comes to abortion when there is danger to the mother's life. Abortion is opposed on the grounds that all life is sacred and at whatever stage in its development, human life must not be destroyed. It is often based on

these religious grounds that countries develop their legal position on abortion. In the Republic of Ireland for example, the Catholic majority population has opposed abortion. It is therefore illegal to have an abortion there. However, Islam teaches that life is sacred and that an abortion can only be carried out if the woman's life is in danger. In this case the mother's life takes precedence over the baby's.

Abortion and the law

In England, Scotland and Wales abortion is regulated by the Abortion Act 1967. It accepts that abortion is justified but only in certain circumstances and before the 24th week of the pregnancy. The Act says that:

- an abortion can legally be carried out if two doctors agree that to continue the pregnancy would put the mother's life at risk or she is at risk of physical or mental injury (which can include serious emotional strain, depression and other forms of mental stress); or,
- two doctors agree that the child is likely to be born with severe mental or physical disability.

An abortion must be carried out before the 24th week of pregnancy, unless a serious risk of life occurs to the mother beyond this period.

If you are under 16 either your parents must give their consent or else the two doctors who agree to the termination must also agree that you are mature enough to understand what their decision means. If the abortion is being carried out after eight weeks then it will be under a general anaesthetic in which case permission may be required from your parents if you are under 16.

The would-be father (whether married or not) has no legal right to prevent the mother from having an abortion. The decision is hers.

The Abortion Act allows doctors and other medical staff to refuse any involvement in the practice of abortion if it is against their conscience. This means that you may want an abortion but your GP will not support you. In a situation like this you can go to another GP for medical advice (you don't have to be registered with that GP if you go for family planning or abortion advice). The GP will then contact your local hospital for an appointment with the second doctor.

Because of the 24-week time factor in terminating a pregnancy and because the number of clinics doing abortions are limited, it is often necessary to travel some distance for an abortion.

In addition to the physical discomfort and pain of an abortion (particularly if it is carried out after 12 weeks) many women have mixed feelings of loss and relief.

Abortion is a taboo subject (one that some people do not like to talk about), it is often more difficult to talk about how you feel to friends

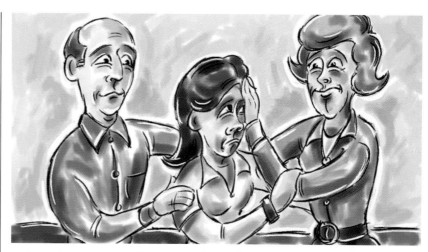

and family. It is a painful emotional experience and you may wish to contact one of the organisations below for support.

Organisations

Abortion Law Reform Association
2-12 Pentonville Road, London, N1 9FP. Tel: 020 7278 5539. Fax: 020 7278 5236. E-mail: choice@alra.org.uk Web site: www.alra.mailbox.co.uk

The Abortion Law Reform Association believes women should be allowed to make up their own minds on abortion, regardless of their circumstances. Women should not be forced by law to rely on the decision of their doctors who are sometimes influenced by moral rather than medical judgement.

British Pregnancy Advisory Service (BPAS)
Austy Manor, Wootten Wawen, Solihull, West Midlands, B95 6BX. Tel: 01564 793225. Helpline: 08457 30 40 30. Web site: www.bpas.org

BPAS Action line open Monday-Friday 8am-9pm, Saturday 8.30am-6pm and Sunday 9.30am-2.30pm

BPAS see many women who are faced with an unplanned pregnancy and find it hard to make a decision about what to do. They are contacted by almost 50,000 women every year.

Brook Publications
165 Grays Inn Road, London, WC1X 8UD. Tel: 020 7833 8488. Fax: 020 7833 8182. Help line: 020 7284 6040. E-mail: info@brookcentres.org.uk Web site: www.brook.org.uk

Brook Advisory Centres has published a booklet, price £2.25,

Abortion – an introduction to the facts available from the address below. Also you can call the Brook Advisory Abortion Helpline.

LIFE (Save the Unborn Child)
Lifehouse, Newbold Terrace, Leamington Spa, Warwickshire, CV32 4EA. Tel: 01926 421587. Help line: 01926 311511. Fax: 01926 336497. E-mail: info@lifeuk.org Web site: www.lifeuk.org

Life is a campaigning group who oppose abortion believing that every unborn child has the right to life. The helpline is available between 9am and 9pm daily.

Marie Stopes International
153-157 Cleveland Street, London, W1P 5PG. Tel: 020 7574 7400. Help line: 0845 300 8090. Fax: 020 7574 7417. E-mail: services@stopes.org.uk Web site: www.mariestopes.org.uk

Marie Stopes International promotes the acceptance of family planning techniques and runs mother and child health and family planning programmes throughout the world.

Support After Termination for Abnormality (SATFA)
73 Charlotte Street, London, W1 1LB. Tel: 020 7439 6124. Help line: 020 7631 0285.

SATFA provides information and support to families who are told that their unborn baby may have an abnormality. They also offer long-term support to parents who choose termination.

- The above information is from the National Youth Agency's web site www.youthinformation.com

© 2003 National Youth Agency

Call for private Scottish abortion clinic

By John Innes

A private abortion clinic might open in Scotland after it emerged that hundreds of women are travelling to England for terminations.

Figures released by the English-based British Pregnancy Advisory Service yesterday reveal that women in Scotland cannot get late abortions and are forced to travel south of the Border.

Ian Jones, chief executive of BPAS, said: 'Our figures show that only 13 per cent of women who come to us for abortions from England and Wales are more than 15 weeks pregnant, compared with 40 per cent of Scottish women.

'The reason for this could be that women in early pregnancy are getting a service in Scotland but those who present later in pregnancy are not. In certain parts of Scotland, they are not geared up to do the later abortions. It gets more difficult after 12 weeks.'

He claimed that the figures meant there was a need for a private clinic in Scotland. But he added that it would not be financially viable to open a centre and that any service would be provided from an existing NHS hospital.

BPAS – which operates 12 clinics in England – has a counselling service in Scotland and has recently moved into NHS premises at the Glasgow-based sexual health clinic, the Sandyford Initiative. Mr Jones said some doctors and nurses would not be prepared to work at the clinic, adding: 'If there were staff willing to do this, late abortions would not be a problem in the first place.

> **'Taking away the physical distance is not going to make late terminations popular, it is just going to make women's lives easier'**

'On the one hand, it is disgraceful that doctors can pick and choose. But if these doctors do not want to treat women for a late abortion then we do not want them treating women.'

Last year 40 per cent of the 218 Scottish women who attended BPAS treatment clinics in England were more than 15 weeks pregnant. Just 13 per cent of the 44,046 women from England and Wales were at a later stage than that.

Times for terminations in Scotland vary across the country. Dr Ursula Bankowska, an associate director of the Sandyford Initiative, backed the calls for a private clinic, saying: 'The decision to have a late termination of pregnancy is a difficult one to make.

'Taking away the physical distance is not going to make late terminations popular, it is just going to make women's lives easier.'

But some anti-abortion campaigners have attacked the move, claiming it is a 'quick-fix' solution. Paul Tully, the general secretary of the Society for the Protection of the Unborn Child, said: 'The BPAS approach is disregarding the whole issue of why women are seeking abortions in these circumstances.

'There are often huge social or personal pressures that are pushing these women towards late abortions.

'Policymakers and health officials should be taking these pressures into account.'

■ The above article is from *The Scotsman*'s web site which can be found at www.scotsman.com

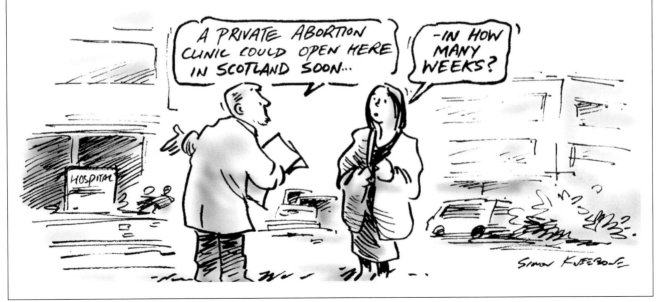

25pc of doctors' practices have anti-abortionist GP

**By Celia Hall,
Medical Editor**

One general practice in four in England includes a family doctor who will not give consent to abortions, according to an official study into teenage pregnancies.

The Teenage Pregnancy Unit at the Department of Health asked all 4,000 practices about GPs' attitudes to abortion and to consultations with teenagers and received responses from 40 per cent.

The survey found that on average 15 per cent of doctors would not see a patient under 16 who was not accompanied by a parent and in some areas 30 per cent of the GPs said they would not see children alone.

The results of the survey were released at a conference last week and the figures may indicate that more doctors are expressing opposition to abortion for social reasons.

Three years ago a survey by Marie Stopes International, the sexual health organisation, found that 18 per cent of doctors were opposed to abortion.

Tony Kerridge, who led the Marie Stopes study, said the figures appeared to show a small rise in opposition to abortion which was significant.

'It can cause delays in women getting an abortion and that makes it more likely that a woman will abort later and that means a more dangerous procedure.'

The Guild of Catholic Doctors said it was 'surprised but delighted' to see that the number of doctors opposed to abortion was so high.

'These doctors do not have to be Catholic to have an objection. A lot of doctors who are not opposed to the principle of abortion are very unhappy to see it used as an extension to contraception,' said Dr Michael Jarmulowicz, the master of the guild.

'They do not feel happy about social abortion, especially when they may see the same woman two or three times,' he said.

'The truth that abortion is destruction of life cannot be denied for ever and it is encouraging that so many doctors are exercising their right to practise by such principles.'

Dr Jarmulowicz said they frequently heard of cases when doctors had 'bluntly' suggested that women consider abortions, usually young unmarried women with unintended pregnancies.

> **'A lot of doctors who are not opposed to the principle of abortion are very unhappy to see it used as an extension to contraception'**

'Such women report they have found such suggestions both offensive and intimidating.'

But he said he was concerned that 15 per cent of GPs said they

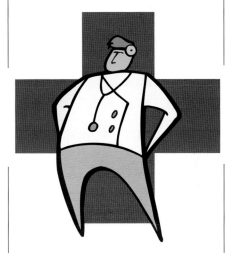

would not see under-16s without their parents.

'There is a difficulty here. If you take cases of sexual abuse by someone in the family a young person may need to see the doctor alone. I would not be happy about a doctor having a blanket ban on seeing patients under 16 alone,' he said.

Alison Hadley, the programme manager of the Government's Teenage Pregnancy Strategy, said the results of the survey showed 'clear gaps in the provision of services'.

Britain has the second highest teenage pregnancy rate in the developed world and the Government is committed to bringing the numbers down.

In 2000 there were 97,600 pregnancies among teenagers in England and Wales of which 395 were among girls under 14, and 8,111 among girls under the age of 16. Pregnancy rates in the under-14s showed no fall over 1999.

In 2001 there were 186,200 abortions in England and Wales compared with 185,400 in the previous year. In 2000, 54 per cent of pregnant girls had abortions compared with 52 per cent in 1999.

A spokesman for the Department of Health said that the 40 per cent response rate to the survey was considered a good response.

'This is the first time we have carried out such an audit. These are preliminary results and are designed to inform our work to improve access to GP services by young people.

'It is known that teenagers seek medical help later in their pregnancies than older women. Doctors are allowed to have conscientious objections to abortion but they must ensure that the patient is referred to another doctor as quickly as possible.

'Practices should have systems in place to ensure a speedy referral to a doctor who does not object,' she said.

■ A young woman under 16 can have an abortion but special rules apply about consent. (p. 1)

■ On average, throughout England and Wales the NHS pays for approximately three-quarters of abortions. (p. 4)

■ Almost 90 per cent of abortions are in the first 12 weeks of pregnancy. Just 1.5 per cent are after 20 weeks. (p. 4)

■ The highest number of abortions is among women aged 20-24. However, a great deal of attention has been focused on teenagers because England and Wales has one of the highest teenage pregnancy rates for 15- 19-year-olds in Western Europe. (p. 5)

■ Abortion of foetuses up to the 24th week of pregnancy is legal in England, Scotland and Wales (in Northern Ireland it is only legal in exceptional circumstances). (p. 6)

■ 180,000 legal abortions are carried out in Britain every year. (p. 6)

■ Abortions must be carried out in a hospital or a clinic approved by the Department of Health. (p. 7)

■ Two doctors need to agree that your abortion is necessary for your mental and/or physical health. (p. 7)

■ Abortion is legal in England, Wales and Scotland but not in Northern Ireland or the Irish Republic where abortion is illegal. (p. 8)

■ There were 4,382 terminations on under-16s in 2000 compared with 3,510 in 1992. (p. 11)

■ Britain has the highest teenage pregnancy rate in Europe. (p. 11)

■ The number of pregnancies among under-16s in 2000 went up by 161 to 8,111 – the first rise in five years. (p. 11)

■ The most common sign of possible pregnancy is a missed period. Other signs are sickness, swollen breasts and passing urine more frequently. (p 12)

■ Over a third of all pregnancies, across the world, are unplanned. (p. 14)

■ When does life begin?
– Not all religions define a particular moment when life begins but some, like Buddhism, Sikhism and Catholicism, teach that life begins at fertilisation – the moment that sperm meets egg. The Roman Catholic Church says that the fertilised egg is a sacred life, with as many rights as a baby, child or adult, and forbids abortion. Amongst Buddhists and Sikhs there is a variety of opinions on the morality of abortion. (p. 14)

■ Two Acts of Parliament, the Abortion Act 1967 and the Human Fertilisation and Embryology Act 1990, regulate the provision of abortion in England, Wales and Scotland. (p. 19)

■ Out of about 173,000 abortions in 1999 (the last year for which statistics are available) 1,813 were for suspected handicap. (p. 24)

■ The Government has vowed to reduce conception rates amongst under-18s by 50% by 2010. (p. 28)

■ Attendance by under-16s at family planning clinics rose by 143.6% between 1992 and 2000. (p. 28)

■ A survey conducted by Marie Stopes International (MSI) in 1999 found that 18% of GPs were opposed to abortion, yet they do not have to declare this objection to patients. (p. 29)

■ Some facts about abortion
– 1 in 5 pregnancies in the UK end in termination
– 90% of all abortions take place in the first 12 weeks of pregnancies
– Over half of all pregnancies in under-16s end in abortion. (p. 36)

■ An abortion must be carried out before the 24th week of pregnancy, unless a serious risk of life occurs to the mother beyond this period. (p. 37)

■ In 2000 there were 97,600 pregnancies among teenagers in England and Wales of which 395 were among girls under 14, and 8,111 among girls under the age of 16. Pregnancy rates in the under-14s showed no fall over 1999. (p. 39)

ADDITIONAL RESOURCES

You might like to contact the following organisations for further information. Due to the increasing cost of postage, many organisations cannot respond to enquiries unless they receive a stamped, addressed envelope.

The Abortion Law Reform Association (ALRA)
2-12 Pentonville Road
London, N1 9FP
Tel: 020 7278 5539
Fax: 020 7278 5236
E-mail: alra@mailbox.co.uk
Web site: www.alra.org.uk
ALRA believes women should be allowed to make up their own minds on abortion, regardless of their circumstances. Women should not be forced by law to rely on the decision of their doctors who are sometimes influenced by moral rather than medical judgement.

British Humanist Association (BHA)
1 Gower Street
London, WC1E 6HD
Tel: 020 7079 3580
Fax: 020 7430 1271
E-mail: info@humanism.org.uk
Web site: www.humanism.org.uk
The BHA exists to support and represent people who seek to live good and responsible lives without religious or superstitious beliefs.

British Pregnancy Advisory Service (BPAS)
Austy Manor, Wootton Wawen
Solihull, West Midlands, B95 6BX
Tel: 01564 793225
Fax: 01564 794935
E-mail: comm.@bpas.org
Web site: www.bpas.org
British Pregnancy Advisory Service supports reproductive choice by advocating and providing high-quality, affordable services to prevent or end unwanted pregnancy with contraception or by abortion. Runs the BPAS Abortion Actionline. To make an appointment phone 08457 304030.

British Victims of Abortion (BVA)
Olympic House, 142 Queens Street
Glasgow, G1 3BU
Tel: 0141 226 5407
Fax: 0141 221 7707
E-mail: info@bvafoundation.org

BVA is committed to exposing the truth of abortion's tragedy in our community. BVA offers counselling on their helpline from 7-10 pm. Tel 0845 603 8501. All calls charged at local rates.

Brook Advisory Centres
Unit 421, Highgate Studios
53-79 Highgate Road
London, NW5 1TL
Tel: 020 7284 6040
Fax: 020 7284 6050
E-mail: admin@brookcentres.org.uk
Web site: www.brook.org.uk
Brook Advisory Centres is the only national voluntary sector provider of free and confidential sexual health advice and services specifically for young people under 25. If you need to speak to someone urgently, you can call the Brook Helpline on 0800 0185 023.

Education for Choice
2-12 Pentonville Road
London, N1 9FP
Tel: 020 7837 7221
Fax: 020 7254 7838
E-mail: efc@efc.org.uk
Web site: www.efc.org.uk
Education for Choice believes that abortion is morally and medically acceptable. Produces a factsheet and education pack which outline their views.

LIFE
LIFE House, Newbold Terrace
Leamington Spa, CV32 4EA
Tel: 01926 421587
Fax: 01926 336497
E-mail: info@lifeuk.org
Web site: www.lifeuk.org
LIFE provides a nationwide care service for pregnant women, unsupported mothers, women with problems relating to pregnancy, fertility or infertility, or suffering from the effects of abortion.

Marie Stopes International
153-157 Cleveland Street
London, W1P 5PG
Tel: 020 7574 7400
Fax: 020 7574 7407

E-mail: service@stopes.org.uk
Web site: www.mariestopes.org.uk, www.likeitis.org.uk and www.abortion-help.co.uk
Marties Stopes International provides sexual and reproductive health information to 33 million worldwide in 38 countries.

National Youth Agency (NYA)
17-23 Albion Street
Leicester, LE1 6GD
Tel: 0116 285 3700
Fax: 0116 285 3777
E-mail: nya@nya.org.uk
Web site: www.nya.org.uk, www.youthinformation.com and www.ypnmagazine.com
The National Youth Agency aims to advance youth work to promote young people's personal and social development, and their voice, influence and place in society.

ProLife Alliance
PO Box 13395
London, SW3 6XE
Tel: 020 7351 9955
Fax: 020 7349 0450
E-mail: info@prolife.org.uk
Web site: www.prolife.org.uk
The ProLife Alliance is Europe's first Pro-Life Political Party. We seek to ensure the right to life of all, the most basic and fundamental human right. To obtain this right, we will use only peaceful and democratic means. We are totally opposed to any form of violent protest.

Society for the Protection of the Unborn Child (SPUC)
Phyllis Bowman House
5-6 St Matthew Street
Westminster
London, SW1P 2JT
Tel: 020 7222 5845
Fax: 020 7222 0630
E-mail: enquiry@spuc.org.uk
Web site: www.spuc.org.uk
SPUC affirms, defends and promotes the existence and value of human life from the moment of conception, and defends and protects human life generally.

INDEX

ACKNOWLEDGEMENTS

The publisher is grateful for permission to reproduce the following material.

While every care has been taken to trace and acknowledge copyright, the publisher tenders its apology for any accidental infringement or where copyright has proved untraceable. The publisher would be pleased to come to a suitable arrangement in any such case with the rightful owner.

Chapter One: The Facts of Abortion
Abortion – the facts, © Brook Advisory Centres, *Public opinions*, © British Pregnancy Advisory Service (BPAS), *Opinions on abortion*, © British Pregnancy Advisory Service (BPAS), *Abortion statistics*, © British Pregnancy Advisory Service (BPAS), *Facts and statistics*, © British Pregnancy Advisory Service (BPAS), *All about abortions*, © Teenage Health Websites Ltd 2003, *Grounds on which abortion is permitted in some countries*, © International Planned Parenthood Federation (IPPF), *Common questions on abortion answered*, © 1999-2003 Pupiline Limited, *Teenage pregnancy*, © Marie Stopes International, *Abortions carried out on under-16s soar*, © The Daily Mail, 2003, *Teenage conception rates*, © Crown copyright is reproduced with the permission of Her Majesty's Stationery Office, *Unwanted pregnancy and abortion*, © The Abortion Law Reform Association (ALRA), *Gestational age*, © Crown copyright is reproduced with the permission of Her Majesty's Stationery Office, *Abortion and religion*, © Education for Choice, *Where do world religions stand on abortion?*, © Education for Choice, *LIFE says attitudes to abortion are changing*, © LIFE, *A non-religious perspective on abortion*, © British Humanist Association (BHA), *Abortion and the law*, © Brook Advisory Centres.

Chapter Two: The Debate
Pro-life or pro-choice?, © 1999-2003 Pupiline Limited, *Hard questions answered*, © LIFE, *Abortion statistics*, © Crown copyright is reproduced with the permission of Her Majesty's Stationery Office, *Widespread ignorance of abortion rights*, © The Abortion Law Reform Association (ALRA), *Opinion poll*, © National Abortion Campaign (NAC), *Abortion FAQs*, © ProLife Alliance, *LIFE mourns 35 years of forgotten fathers*, © LIFE, *Men too*, © British Pregnancy Advisory Service (BPAS), *Questions men ask us*, © British Pregnancy Advisory Service (BPAS), *The ages of women having abortions*, © Crown copyright is reproduced with the permission of Her Majesty's Stationery Office, *Teenage pregnancies*, © SPUC, *One in three*, © Guardian Newspapers Limited 2003, *Marital status*, © Crown copyright is reproduced with the permission of Her Majesty's Stationery Office, *Manifestations of post-abortion trauma*, © British Victims of Abortion (BVA), *Tough life choices*, © Guardian Newspapers Limited 2003, *Why abortion is bad for your mental health*, © Telegraph Group Limited, London 2003, *Coping with termination*, © 2003 National Youth Agency, *Call for private Scottish abortion clinic*, © 2003 The Scotsman, *25 pc of doctors' practices have anti-abortionist GP*, © Telegraph Group Limited, London 2003.

Photographs and illustrations:
Pages 1, 9, 29, 37: Pumpkin House; pages 4, 12, 24, 35: Bev Aisbett; pages 6, 14, 17, 19, 22, 38: Simon Kneebone.

Craig Donnellan
Cambridge
September, 2003